ELLIE HERMAN'S

PILATES SPRINGBOARD

ALSO BY ELLIE HERMAN

Pilates for Dummies

Pilates Mat

Pilates Reformer

Pilates Springboard

Pilates Cadillac

Pilates Wunda Chair

Pilates Arc & Barrel

Pilates Props Workbook

Pilates Workbook on the Ball

ELLIE HERMAN'S

PILATES SPRINGBOARD

BY ELLIE HERMAN
ELLIE HERMAN BOOKS, BROOKLYN

Published in the United States by
Ellie Herman Books
788A Union Street
Brooklyn, NY 11215
www.elliehermanpilates.com

ISBN 978-1-4675-0207-8

Ellie Herman, author
Susi May, co-author
Elizabeth Gand, copy editor
Jenny Belluomini, copy editor

Design & composition by SeMe Sung, Stephen Nichols, & Margaret Banda.

Printed in Canada by Transcontinental Printing.

Please Note:
This book has been written and published strictly for informational purposes, and in no way should be used as a substitute for consultation with Pilates and/or health care professionals. You should not consider educational material herein to be the practice of medicine or to replace consultation with a physician or other medical practitioner. The author and publisher are providing you with information in this work so that you can have the knowledge and can choose, at your own risk, to act on that knowledge. The author and publisher also urge all readers to be aware of their health status and to consult health care professionals before beginning any health program.

This book is dedicated to Phil Cusick, who was an inspiration and co-designer for the Springboard, and a dear, dear friend.

TABLE OF CONTENTS

LEG SPRINGS

THE PILATES SPRINGBOARD PROTOTYPE
DESIGNED BY ELLIE HERMAN & PHIL CUSICK

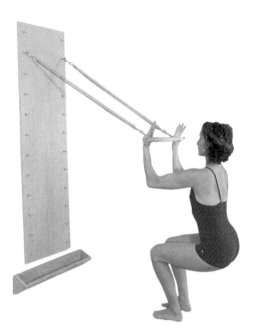

The photos of the Springboard in this book were taken with Ellie on the original Springboard prototype.

A space saving and affordable piece of resistance equipment based on the Cadillac (or Trap Table) which gives you a full-body workout.

The **Pilates Springboard** consists of a six-foot rectangular wooden board with eyelets placed on either side at six-inch increments and a dowel at the bottom to use for arm or foot support. It comes with:
- two arm springs with neoprene handles
- two leg springs, with cotton loops
- one wooden roll-down bar

It comes with a 45 minute flow workout DVD which takes you through a warm-up, core strengthening, upper body and lower body conditioning program. Some of the exercises are from classic Pilates repertoire, and others are original exercises developed especially for the Springboard by master Pilates teacher Ellie Herman.

The **Pilates Springboard** is bolted into studs for support, taking up no floor space. This makes it perfect for an extra room, a home gym, garage, attic, or basement. For those with gyms or Pilates studios, you can affordably mount several Springboards along a wall and offer challenging Pilates group equipment classes without moving heavy equipment or taking up valuable storage space.

Manufactured by **Balanced Body**, the leader in Pilates equipment.

Springboard vs. Reformer
Springboard springs differ from the Reformer pulley system in at least two important ways. First, with springs, each arm or leg has its own separate resistance as opposed to the Reformer, where the arms or legs share the resistance. With springs, therefore, a dominant arm or leg will become noticeable where it may not be on the Reformer. Also springs are more unstable; they have an uneven pull as opposed to the smooth pulley system on the Reformer. Springs are more conditioning for this reason as well as being better for teaching more advanced stabilization.

THE PILATES SPRINGBOARD
BY BALANCED BODY

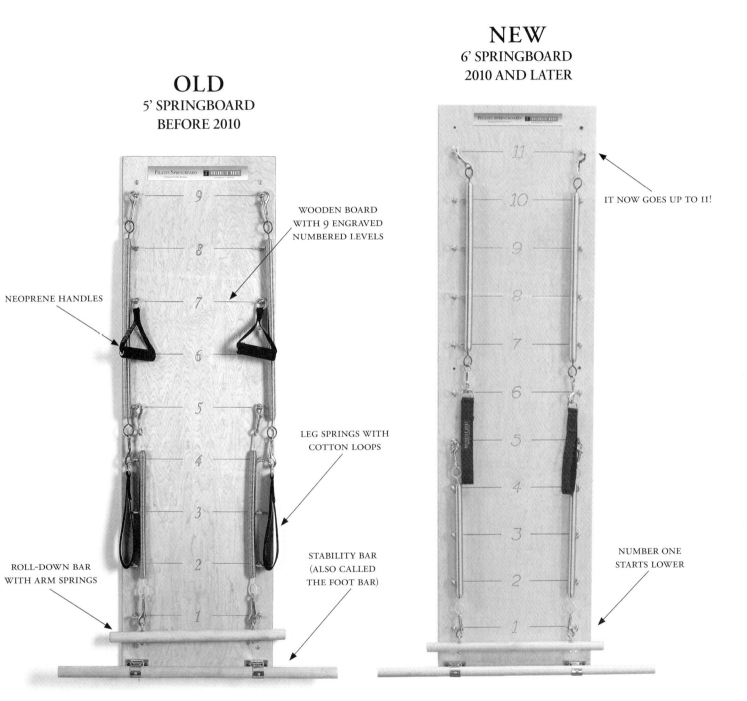

NEW
6' SPRINGBOARD
2010 AND LATER

OLD
5' SPRINGBOARD
BEFORE 2010

WOODEN BOARD
WITH 9 ENGRAVED
NUMBERED LEVELS

IT NOW GOES UP TO 11!

NEOPRENE HANDLES

LEG SPRINGS WITH
COTTON LOOPS

ROLL-DOWN BAR
WITH ARM SPRINGS

STABILITY BAR
(ALSO CALLED
THE FOOT BAR)

NUMBER ONE
STARTS LOWER

Since the numbers on the new Springboard start lower you will need to adjust your spring settings one and possibly two eyebolts higher for every exercise if you have the newer Springboard.

AN INTRODUCTION TO ELLIE HERMAN

I discovered Pilates many moons ago when I was a professional dancer and choreographer in San Francisco circa 1988. Needless to say, my work with *The Flying Buttresses* feminist performance troupe did not garner enough cash to support my bohemian lifestyle in the Bay Area. And being 22, full of hubris, and an experience junky to boot, I did what every self-respecting young woman in my position would do—I became a professional wrestler. But my career as "Ruth Less" was cut short; during a tag team match one squat, tough cookie tried to take me down, but I stayed my ground—only to hear a loud "snapping" sound. My anterior cruciate ligament. Torn. For good. As I lay on the mat, I cursed myself; how could I be so stupid? I figured my dance career was over for sure.

Enter Pilates. I ventured to St. Francis Hospital in San Francisco where they have a whole Dance Medicine department dedicated to Pilates-based rehabilitation, and was put under the care of Elizabeth Larkham. After six months of rehabilitation, I returned to dancing only to realize that Pilates had not only allowed me to return to jumping, leaping, and twirling, it had actually improved my technique, control, balance, and core strength.

I then moved to New York City, where I enrolled in the MFA program in dance at New York University, and I took morning Pilates Mat classes with Kathy Grant, one of Joseph Pilates' original disciples. Kathy taught me how depth and creativity could be brought to the Pilates Method—while helping to relieve the mounting hip pain I was experiencing due to daily ballet classes. I dropped out of the Master's program, but Kathy Grant inspired me to pursue Pilates teacher training—which I did with Steve Giordano and Romana Kryzanowska (another of Joe Pilates' original students).

I returned to San Francisco in 1992 and continued my Pilates studies with Jennifer Stacey and Carol Appel of Body Kinetics. The following year I opened my own studio in my live/work loft in the Mission

district of San Francisco. The studio expanded so much over the years that we moved to a bigger building, with two full floors dedicated to Pilates-based fitness, rehabilitation, teacher training, continuing education, and complementary medicine. As Pilates gained popularity, my business grew, and I opened a second studio in Oakland, California, in 2001.

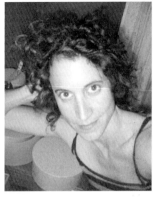

ELLIE HERMAN

My hunger for knowledge led me to earn a Master of Science degree in Acupuncture & Chinese Herbal Medicine at the American College of Traditional Chinese Medicine in San Francisco in 2000.

I started to miss my family and the East Coast edge, so I moved to Brooklyn and opened my third studio in Park Slope in October of 2005. I then opened a second studio in Park Slope in 2010 called the Annex, where we offer group classes in all kinds of mind body fitness. I sold my California studios and am now solely based in Brooklyn.

As part of my ongoing interest in Pilates innovation, I designed a new piece of Pilates equipment called the *Pilates Springboard*. The Springboard is an inexpensive and space-saving variation of the Wall Unit/Cadillac which is now being manufactured by Balanced Body.

Although Pilates is a fabulous system that can correct and rehabilitate a plethora of physical ailments, it doesn't always translate to standing and gait. Since an active person takes over 5,000 steps a day, I became obsessed with the notion of how our gait reinforces postural habits. With the help of the lovely and brilliant Nancy Myers (the former VP of Ellie Herman Studios, who can see a gait abnormality a mile away), I developed a system that combines Pilates and walking called *Walk-ilates.*^{SM}

Please check out my blog on my website, **www.elliehermanpilates.com** for the latest news on my studios and other adventures in Pilates. I am available for workshops and teacher trainings. Contact me at **ellie@elliehermanpilates.com**.

THE SKINNY ON MR. PILATES

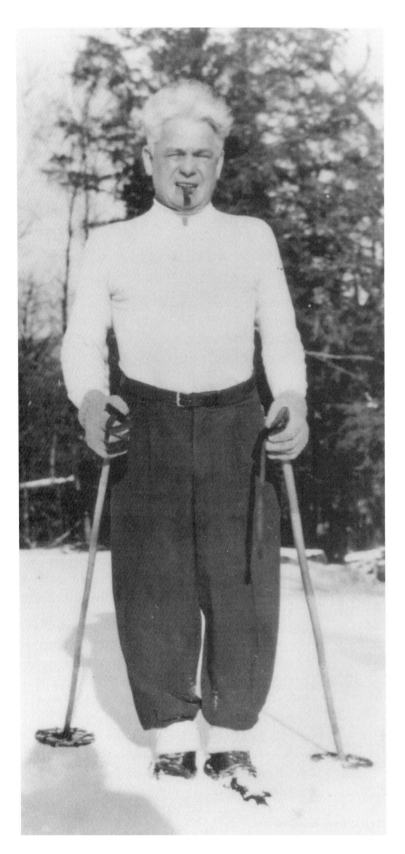

Joseph Hubertus Pilates was born in Germany in 1880, and as a young man suffered from asthma and poor health. Over his lifetime, he overcame his frailties and became an accomplished athlete—an avid skier, diver, gymnast, yogi, and pugilist.

Mr. Pilates was a visionary who had overarching ideas about how to be a healthy happy human. He first developed a series of exercises to be done on a mat designed to build abdominal strength and overall body control. He then invented various pieces of equipment to enhance the results of his expanding repertoire of exercises. The apocryphal story goes that Joseph Pilates was a nurse stationed in an English internment camp during WWI, and he had the bright idea to rig springs above hospital beds, which allowed patients to rehabilitate their injuries and to exercise while lying on their backs. This bed-like set-up later evolved into the Cadillac, one of the main pieces of Pilates equipment.

In 1923 Joseph Pilates emigrated to the United States, settling in New York City, where he opened a studio on Eighth Avenue in Manhattan and started training and rehabilitating professional dancers including George Balanchine and Martha Graham.

In his book *Return to Life*, Joseph Pilates lays out a whole regime to improve overall health, including of course, the classical Pilates Mat exercises, with Joe himself pictured going through the whole series (worth seeing!). He originally called his method "Contrology" and only after he taught his method to others was it referred to as "Pilates." In his book he states, "[Contrology] develops the body uniformly, corrects wrong postures, restores physical vitality, invigorates the mind, and elevates the spirit."

Over his lifetime, Pilates invented over 20 contraptions some of which look a little like medieval torture devices—constructed of wood and metal piping, using a variable combination of pulleys, straps, bars, boxes, and springs. The total Pilates repertoire consists of over 500 exercises, including Pilates Mat, Reformer, Cadillac, Wunda Chair, Spine Corrector, Ladder Barrel, and Tower.

THE PILATES LINEAGE

The original Eighth Avenue Pilates studio in Manhattan bore the first generation of Pilates teachers: Romana Kryzanowska, Kathy Grant, Ron Fletcher, Eve Gentry, Carola Trier, Mary Bowen, and Bruce King. Some of these protégés branched out and opened studios around the country, while others stayed in New York City. Romana remained in Joe's original studio until after his death. Kathy Grant, who passed away in May 2010, in a small studio above the NYU dance department, where I was fortunate enough to have been graced by her presence. For the last 50 years, the Pilates Method has been passed down through many more generations of teachers and the Method has transformed a great deal along the way. Many modern Pilates teachers now bring their own insights to improve the original, while others cling to the notion of a "pure" Pilates which, in their mind should not be trifled with! In my opinion, if Mr. Pilates was an innovator, and within his own lifetime changed and evolved his repertoire and invented new contraptions, why shouldn't we?

WHAT EXACTLY IS PILATES?

Pilates exercises as a whole develop strong abdominal, back, butt, and deep postural muscles to support the skeletal system and act as what Pilates called the "powerhouse" of the body. The Pilates Method works to strengthen the center, lengthen the spine, increase body awareness, build muscle tone and gain flexibility. The Pilates Method is also an excellent rehabilitation system for back, knee, hip, shoulder and repetitive stress injuries. Pilates addresses the body as a whole, correcting the body's asymmetries and chronic weaknesses to prevent re-injury and bring the body back into balance.

EIGHT PRINCIPLES OF PILATES

Joseph Pilates' book, *Return to Life,* maps out the eight important principles that underlie the Pilates Method. These concepts are the backbone of the Pilates Method.

CONTROL

A fundamental rule when doing Pilates: Control your body's every movement! This rule applies not only to the exercises themselves but also to transitions between exercises, how you get on and off the equipment, and your overall attention to detail while working out. When doing Mat exercises, Control comes into play with the attack and ending of each movement. When the body puts on the brakes in a controlled manner, it is training the muscles to work as they lengthen. This is called eccentric muscle contraction, which builds long and flexible muscles. Also, when focusing on Control of a movement, the body is forced to recruit helper muscles (we call these synergists), which are usually smaller than the main muscles. When many muscles work together to do one movement, or when muscles work synergistically, the body as a whole develops greater balance and co-ordination. Also, the big muscles won't bulk up because they don't have to do all the work by themselves. Thus we become a long and lean machine. Once your body learns to move with Control you will feel more confident doing all kinds of things from skiing that advanced run, to tango dancing, or to climbing a ladder to get up to that rocking roof deck party.

BREATH

Most people do not utilize their full lung capacity. Shallow breathing is an unfortunate side effect of a sedentary and stressful life. Also, as a Pilates instructor it's painful to see how people often hold their breath when performing a new or difficult task. I often have to tell my clients to exhale, because otherwise they won't! Some people will actually get out of breath during a new exercise merely because they haven't exhaled. When you hold your breath, you tense

muscles that can ultimately exacerbate improper posture and reinforce tension habits. That is why consistent Breathing is essential to flowing movement and proper muscle balance. As with yoga, Breathing is an essential part of the Pilates Method and distinguishes it from other exercise forms.

Every Pilates exercise has a specific Breathing pattern assigned to it. Breathing while moving is not always an easy assignment, but when accomplished, beautiful things can happen. Focused Breath can help maximize the body's ability to stretch, and through this release of tension you will gain optimal body Control. Deep inhalation and full exhalation also exercise the lungs and increase lung capacity, bringing deep relaxation as a pleasant side effect.

FLOWING MOVEMENT

If you look at photographs of Pilates exercises, you might notice the similarity to many yoga postures. But unlike yoga, we do not hold positions in Pilates—instead we Flow from one movement to another. When doing a Pilates workout, you want to Flow and move freely during the movement phase and finish with control and precision. Flowing Movement integrates the nervous system, the muscles, and the joints, and trains the body to move smoothly and evenly.

PRECISION

Precision is similar to Control with the added element of spatial awareness. When attacking any movement you must know exactly where that movement starts and ends. All Pilates exercises have precise definitions of where the body should be at all times: the angle of the legs, the placement of the elbows, the positioning of the head and neck, even what the fingers are doing! The little things count in Pilates.

CENTERING

Sometimes after a long day of training clients, I can hear a tape running inside my head that says, "pull the navel to the spine...." Why? Because I have repeated this mantra all day to cue my clients to scoop in their bellies. All exercises should be done with the deep abdominals engaged to ensure proper Centering. Most Pilates exercises focus on developing abdominal strength either directly or indirectly. Even when performing an exercise that focuses on strengthening the arm muscles, you should keep your Abdominal Scoop, keep your shoulders pulling down the back, and perhaps even squeeze your butt. All these actions promote Centering and core muscle strength. No exercise should be done to the detriment of core stabilization. In other words, if your spine moves like a noodle when it should be a rock-hard *Plank*, then you are not allowed to progress to the next level of an exercise.

STABILITY

Pilates exercises utilize the concept of Stability—whether it be torso Stability, shoulder Stability or ankle Stability—which is the key to health for your spine and joints. After an injury, there will generally be instability in the affected area. The first thing you want to do is learn to stabilize the injured part so as to prevent re-injury and to allow the healing process to begin. Thus Pilates is one of the safest forms of exercise to do after injury. Pilates will also prevent injury, for if you have Stability in your torso and joints, you are much less likely to injure yourself in the first place.

RANGE OF MOTION

Range of Motion is a phrase used by medical professionals to describe the movement of a joint. For instance, the Range of Motion of your shoulder joint is defined by how high you can raise your arm in front of you, behind you, etc. Range of Motion can be affected by the length or tightness in your muscles and other tissues such as ligaments and fascia (connective tissue). Basically, Range of Motion is just another way of describing flexibility. If you lack flexibility in your joints or spine, then Pilates can increase Range of Motion. But if you have too much Range of Motion, which causes instability in the joints and spine, then Pilates exercises will teach you how to stabilize those areas. This is how Pilates brings balance to the body. It is important to understand how to limit your Range of Motion if you lack Stability because this will help to prevent injury in the future.

OPPOSITION

Down to go up. Up to go down. When teaching Pilates I often use imagery that uses the concept of Opposition to enhance the form of the exercise. For instance, when doing a Roll Down, which starts seated and upright, I'll always say, "imagine you have a golden string lifting you up from the back of the top of your head as you roll down your spine...." This gives the client the idea to lift up really tall before flexing and rolling back. Basically, going up as they go down. This lengthens the spine and takes the compression out of flexing the spine. This is essential to keeping the spine healthy and injury free. Opposition can be used in many ways to get better form from your clients.

ELLIE'S NINTH PRINCIPLE: BODY AWARENESS

Most of us never learned how to live in our bodies. We don't really know how to sit, stand or walk properly, and we certainly don't know how to fix ourselves once we are broken. Pilates can teach you all this. That's why I call it "high exercise"—because it teaches us the fundamentals of how to take care of our spine, joints, and muscles. It teaches us how to not hurt ourselves and how to get the most longevity from our physical beings.

Many clients have told me that they can hear my voice in their head saying things like, "...relax your shoulders, lengthen through the back of your neck, scoop your belly in."

If you suffer from pain because of faulty postural habits that you aren't even aware of, after a few good sessions with a competent Pilates instructor you will be pleasantly surprised by how fast a newfound awareness can affect a positive change in your body.

ELLIE HERMAN'S PILATES ALPHABET

Just as every word can be broken down into letters, so can every Pilates exercise be broken down into discrete parts. The Pilates alphabet is my way to facilitate the learning process and demystify even the most complex Pilates exercises. Almost every advanced exercise contains basic movements that repeat over and over in the repertoire.

ABDOMINAL SCOOP

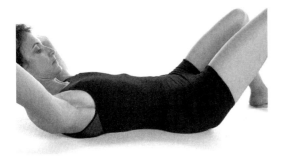

"Pull the navel in toward the spine...." I've probably said that phrase over a million times in my life. It is the first, middle and last cue in the Pilates Method. The Abdominal Scoop can be done anywhere and at any time, and frankly it should be done as much as possible. Anatomically, "the scoop" engages your deepest abdominal muscles, which function to hold in your viscera and, when contracted, decrease the diameter of the abdominal wall. The Abdominal Scoop works a lot like a drawstring around a pair of sweat pants when pulled taut. You have four layers of abdominal muscles; your deepest one is called the transversus abdominis. The second and third layers are called your internal and external obliques. And the most superficial abdominal layer is called your rectus abdominis. The rectus (as we call it in the biz) is a workaholic muscle and will do all the work if you let it. The Abdominal Scoop, or "navel to spine" image is meant to bring in the deeper three layers, which work to compress the abdominal wall and help support

the back. In every exercise you want to be using your Abdominal Scoop to get the most profound results possible. Pooching is the opposite of scooping, so no pooching allowed!

BALANCE POINT

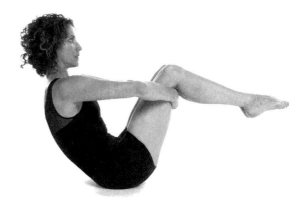

Balance Point, in my vocabulary, is both a position and a fundamental Pilates Mat exercise. As a position, it where you begin and end the rolling exercises on the Mat, and it is also the place you arrive at the top of the *Teaser*. You can practice *Balance Point* by sitting up with your knees bent, holding on to the backs of your thighs. Roll back slightly behind your tailbone, pull your belly in, and lift your feet off the floor. In order to maintain your balance and stop yourself from rolling backward, you must engage and pull in your deep abdominal muscles and slightly round the low back. This teaches you that to balance with ease, you must engage your deep abdominals.

BRIDGE

Bridge is a both a basic position in Pilates that we come in and out of, as well as a beginning level exercise on the Mat and the ball. In kinesiological terms, a *Bridge* is extension of the hips. In lay terms, this means lifting your hips up off the floor, using your butt and hamstrings. I want to point out that a *Bridge* should be done from the hip extensors (butt and hamstrings) and not from the back muscles. Therefore when doing a *Bridge* you must keep your spine neutral (or even slightly flexed) and make sure not to extend (arch) the spine! This is not Yoga!

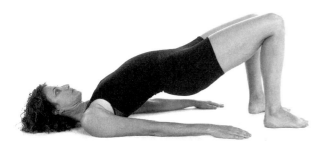

CORRECT BRIDGE: THE BACK IS NEUTRAL

INCORRECT BRIDGE: THE BACK IS HYPEREXTENDED

C-CURVE

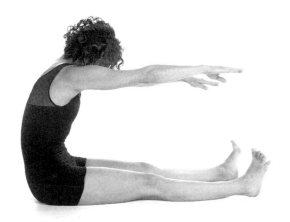

DOOR FRAME ARMS

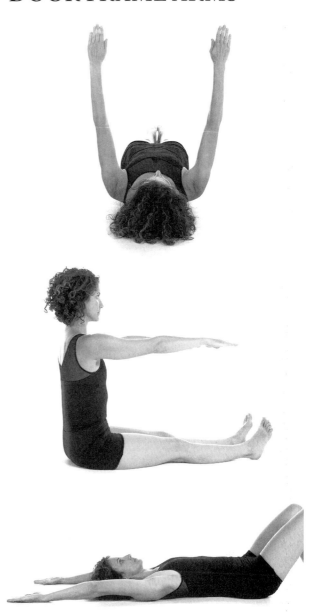

DOOR FRAME ARMS: 3 WAYS

Martha Graham, the mother of Modern Dance, introduced spinal flexion, (or what she termed "the contraction") which revolutionized dance. It was a primal, dark, and oh-so-human movement. Joe Pilates worked with Graham in his Eighth Avenue studio and, I suspect, learned a couple of tricks from her. (Who knows—maybe she learned them from him?) The C-Curve is rounding of the back, or flexion of the spine. The "C" is meant to describe the shape of the back after you scoop in your belly. This shape should always be initiated by your deep Abdominal Scoop and should provide a lovely stretch for your spine. Many Pilates exercises use the C-Curve.

Arms are straight, shoulder distance apart, making the shape of the outer frame of a door. This describes the shape of your arms in many Pilates exercises, whether your arms are above your head, by your sides when lying supine on the floor, or supporting you in a *Plank* position.

HIP UP

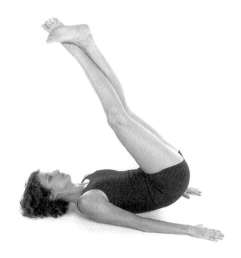

The name says it all. Lie on your back with your legs up, your knees bent, and your Door Frame Arms down by your sides. Rock back and lift your hips up by using your low Abdominal Scoop. The *Hip Up* works your lower abdominals and can be very challenging for those with a weak low abdominals, a tight back, or a large butt!

LEVITATION

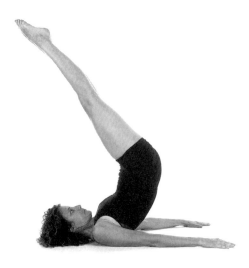

When you combine a *Hip Up* with hip extension, you get Levitation. Try it if you like: lie on your back, lift up your hips with your Abdominal Scoop, and at the top of the *Hip Up*, squeeze your butt. You'll feel your hips levitate, rising perceptibly higher, as if the hand of the Pilates Goddess came down and lifted your hips magically and effortlessly off the floor.

PILATES ABDOMINAL POSITIONING

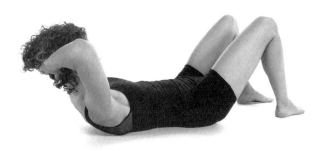

The Pilates Abdominal Positioning is my way to describe the placement of the upper body when performing many of the supine Pilates floor exercises. When lying on your back (supine), lift your head off the floor just high enough so that the bottom tips of your shoulder blades are either just touching or just off the floor. Imagine that the base of the sternum is anchored to the floor and the back of the neck and upper back are stretching around that anchor. Make sure to keep a space the size of a tangerine under your chin (see page 18); you are not meant to over-stretch the back of your neck. It is essential to maintain this position when performing abdominal exercises. If you allow the head to drop back you will begin to feel fatigue in the neck and you will not be using your abdominals as much. The upper abdominals should be working to maintain this position, and that's where you should feel the burn.

PILATES "V" (PILATES FIRST POSITION)

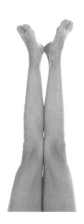

First Position in dance means standing with your legs together and turned out from the hip, knees facing away from each other, and feet making a "V" shape. The Pilates "V" is very much the same except you never want to force the turn out. Your feet should be making a small "V" shape, like a slice of pie, a nice small Pilates-sized slice. In Pilates we use this First Position in many exercises because external rotation of the hips engages the gluteus maximus and the inner thigh muscles, which helps to stabilize the pelvis and spine. (See Parallel vs. Turn Out in the General Movement Vocabulary section.) But lately I prefer to do most exercises in Parallel because it is more functional. The exercises where I continue to use Turn-Out are those that are not functional, like Levitation ie. Magician series on the Springboard, where the use of the gluts helps with pelvic stability and protects the spine from injury.

SERAPE

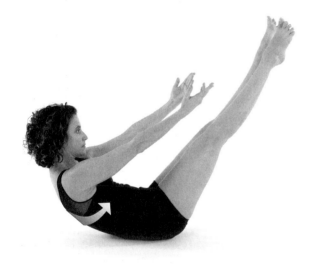

A Serape is a shawl that wraps around your body from the back to the front. This is an image we use in my studios to describe the connection of the shoulder blades pulling down the back as you lift your arms forward—as in *Teaser*. The fibers of the serratus anterior and the obliques interdigitate, connecting the back to the front. Think: "down to go up" as you lift your arms, as if they emanate from the upper back.

ROSEBUD

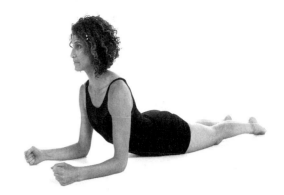

CORRECT NECK PLACEMENT: ROSEBUD ATOP STEM

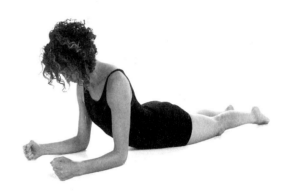

BROKEN BUD: TOO MUCH FLEXION

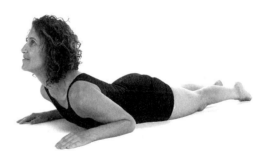

BROKEN BUD: TOO MUCH EXTENSION

In every bunch of roses, there always seems to be one with a broken bud—that sad rose that hangs down from the stem. If you imagine your head as the bud and your spine as the stem in a healthy unbroken rose, then in any movement of your spine, your head will follow and continue the curve of the spine without a break. When you move your head in a "faulty" sequence (say, when you come up into a *Swan* or perform back extension from lying on your belly), your head can look like a broken bud; that is, your neck is bent at a greater angle than the rest of your spine. We want no broken buds in Pilates—only healthy long-stem roses.

SQUEEZE A TANGERINE

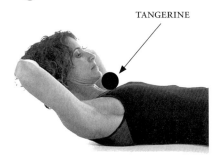

TANGERINE

This is an image that describes the sequencing of your head as you lift it off the floor in flexion. First you should do a small head nod, bring the chin in toward the chest (but don't "juice your tangerine"—keep a small space under your chin) before lifting your head off the floor. The muscle sequencing should be: first your deep neck flexors should fire to nod your head down slightly, then the abdominals lift the head off the mat. The tangerine is the perfect size to imagine the correct distance your chin should be from your chest when holding your Pilates Abdominal Positioning.

TABLE TOP LEGS

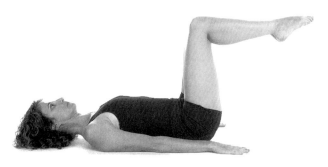

Table Top Legs describes the position of your legs when you are lying supine (on your back), with the knees and feet up off the floor, inner thighs pulling together, knees bent at a 90° angle, and the thighs at a 90° angle to the floor.

STACKING THE SPINE

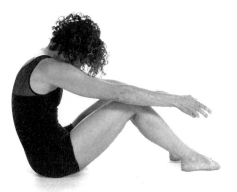

STACKING THE SPINE 1

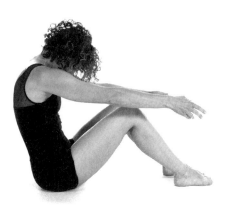

STACKING THE SPINE 2

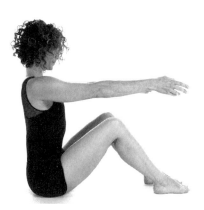

STACKING THE SPINE 3

Stacking the Spine is the ending to a few exercises in the Pilates Method. Stacking the Spine teaches spinal articulation as well as how to sit up vertically. It is a way to sit up or stand erect from a flexed position. Stacking the Spine teaches sequencing from the tail to the head. You start usually from a C-Curve and then stack up from the base of the spine, one vertebra at a time, with the head staying heavy and dropped until the very end. The spine should be completely vertical at the end, with the natural curves of the back in place. (This can be practiced against a wall to better feel the vertical alignment of the spine.)

THORACIC SHELF

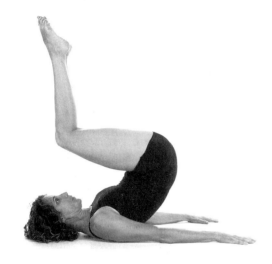

CORRECT NECK PLACEMENT:
BALANCE BETWEEN YOUR SHOULDER BLADES
ON YOUR "THORACIC SHELF"

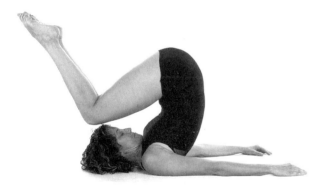

INCORRECT NECK PLACEMENT:
DON'T ROLL ONTO YOUR NECK

This describes the place you want to balance when you are doing all supine inversions that require you to roll onto your upper back. In other words, balance on your shoulder blades, not your neck. This is difficult for people with a tight thoracic spine.

GENERAL MOVEMENT VOCABULARY

ARTICULATION

This is another word for Range of Motion. We use this word mainly when referring to moving the spine one vertebra at a time while rounding down to the Mat, as opposed to coming down in one piece.

ASIS (ANTERIOR SUPERIOR ILIAC SPINE)

ASIS refers to the bony protrusions at the front the pelvis, palpable in standing and even more visible when supine. They are great bony landmarks to monitor pelvic alignment.

CONTINUOUS BREATHING

Breathe by inhaling and exhaling in an even rhythm rather than coordinating the breath with specific body movements.

EXTENSION

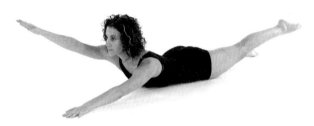

EXTENSION OF THE SPINE, HIPS, KNEES AND ANKLES

Technically, Extension is a movement that brings a part of the body backward from its normal anatomical position, but we also use Extension to mean *to straighten*—as in "straighten your knee." It can also mean *to lengthen* or *stretch*, as in "extend you arms and legs long on the mat." Extension of the spine means the spine is arched back, opening the belly, while the head or tail move backward or toward each other; the *Swan* movement is a perfect example of this principle.

FLEXION

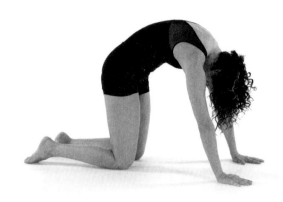

FLEXION OF THE SPINE, SHOULDERS, HIPS, AND KNEES

Flexion is the opposite of Extension: it's a movement that brings a part of the body forward from its normal anatomical position. It also means *to bend*, as in "flex your knee." Flexion of the spine is the movement that brings the head forward (closer) to the pelvis or vice versa; the C-Curve or any abdominal curving is a good example.

PARALLEL VS. TURN OUT

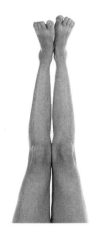

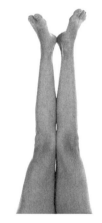

PARALLEL LEGS
TURNED OUT LEGS; PILATES FIRST POSITION

If you've ever taken a modern dance class then you probably have heard the terms Parallel legs and Turned Out legs. Simply put, Parallel means your legs are neutral, with knees facing forward as most of us do naturally when we stand. Turn Out or external rotation of the hips means your knees and feet are facing away from each other and your leg bones are laterally rotated in the hip socket. All ballet dance is done in Turn Out, while modern dance often has movements that use the legs in Parallel. In Pilates, we do many exercises in Turn Out (see Pilates "V" from the Pilates Alphabet). Why Turn Out? Because it engages both the butt and inner thighs, and can help stabilize your pelvis during certain exercises. The longer I teach, the more I move away from Turn Out as the default position. I do most exercises in Parallel since it works the inner thighs in a more functional way—connecting to the core.

PRONE

This term means lying on your belly.

THE POWERHOUSE

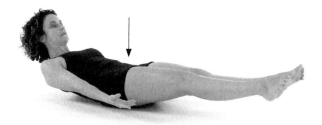

THE POWERHOUSE

The Powerhouse is a term that came from Joe Pilates himself, used today mostly by old school New York trainers. The abdominals, butt, and inner thigh muscles, when working together, constitute the Powerhouse. This is where many of the Pilates exercises initiate when done in the old school style of Turn Out and Flat Back. It is also the area that is challenged in many exercises. In the old days, these muscles were thought to be the main stabilizing muscles of the body, but we now know that the core musculature is what stabilizes the spine. Please refer to page 28.

RELEVÉ / HIGH HEEL FEET

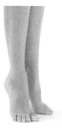

The foot is positioned so the weight of the foot is on the ball and toes. The ankle is in plantar flexion but the toes are in dorsiflexion.

SUPINE

This is a term that simply means lying on your back. Think: spine (Supine with the "u" taken out).

TORSO STABILITY

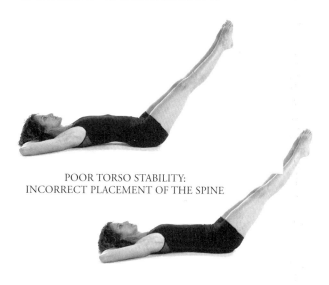

POOR TORSO STABILITY: INCORRECT PLACEMENT OF THE SPINE

STRONG TORSO STABILITY: CORRECT PLACEMENT OF THE SPINE WITH NEUTRAL CURVES AND NO EXCESSIVE LUMBAR CURVATURE

Torso Stability is accomplished mainly by abdominal strength and is one of the most important concepts in the Pilates Method. Most Pilates exercises require you to maintain a stable torso while the arms or legs move. Again, the abdominals are responsible for keeping the spine still while forces are moving around it. So when you are doing one of these Stability exercises (and you can tell if it is a Stability exercise if you hold the torso in one place for the duration of the exercise), simply think to yourself "don't move"—this is the essence of Stability.

NEUTRAL SPINE & THE CORE

Neutral Spine is one of the most subtle, yet powerful principles in the Pilates Alphabet. When the spine is neutral you have three spinal curves (cervical, thoracic, and lumbar) which function to absorb shock when running, jumping, or simply walking around town. And ultimately if you live in Neutral Spine, you will be putting the least amount of stress on the muscles and bones. That's the beauty of perfect posture: it actually feels better. We want to maintain and reinforce these natural curves and that is why we often work in Neutral Spine when performing stability exercises in Pilates.

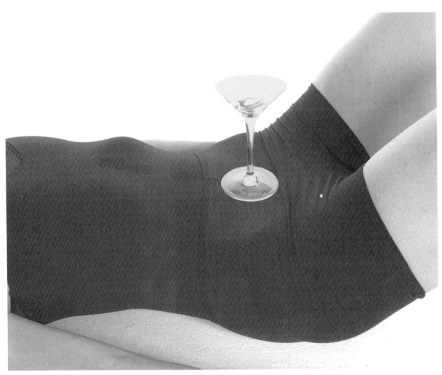

FINDING NEUTRAL SPINE—NOT AS EASY AS YOU MIGHT THINK!

I spend the first two to three hours in my teacher trainings explaining and demonstrating how to find Neutral Spine with all the students. This is not a simple task, and it requires you to use your anatomy knowledge, proprioceptive skills and intuition as an instructor. Sorry, but there is no protocol here!

The first place to start is to find Neutral Pelvis, which is easily defined by objective measures: the ASIS (the hip bones) and the pubic bone form a triangle which forms a plane that should be parallel to the floor when lying down. You (or your client) can feel these bony landmarks with your fingers when supine, and this triangle of bones, when neutral, should create a flat table that could support a filled-to-the-brim double martini. When your pelvis is neutral, your martini will be perfectly balanced. If your pelvis is tilted forward (anterior pelvic tilt—arching your low back too much off the floor) or tilted back (posterior pelvic tilt—flattening your low back onto the floor), your

martini will spill in one of those directions. When lying supine in Neutral Pelvis you should have two areas that do not touch the floor beneath you: your neck and your low back (cervical and lumbar spine, respectively).

NEUTRAL PELVIS VS. NEUTRAL SPINE

When lying supine, the spine does not act the same way as it does when standing, so you need to make adjustments accordingly.

Some people may find, when supine, that being in Neutral Pelvis puts their lumbar or thoracic spine into too much extension, and they will feel uncomfortable in this position. Why? Because even though their pelvis is neutral, their *spine* is not neutral—they have too much lumbar or thoracic curve and their back extensor muscles are contracted. This is not comfortable!

Neutral Spine cannot be measured objectively like Neutral Pelvis since everyone has different spinal curvatures, skeletal structures, and musculature. These put the spine into different positions when lying down. Even the size of someone's derriere will change how the spine configures itself when supine. But as an instructor, your goal is to help your client find the optimal position of the spine and pelvis that allows the back muscles to remain relaxed while supine, while still maintaining some curvature.

Touch your clients

To help clients find Neutral Spine, trainers can put their hands underneath their client's lumbar spine to feel for too much space—your hand should not be able to slide all the way under the back to the other side. There should be a small space under the lumbar spine (not a huge one!). Also your hand should not be able to slide under their thoracic spine (ribcage). If you notice that the ribcage is lifted, cue your client to drop and release the ribcage down to the mat by engaging the upper abdominals. The thoracic spine should be making complete contact with the mat.

Trainers should also feel for contracted spinal extensor muscles—these muscles should stay relaxed. Ask your client if they feel comfortable—believe me, they'll know!

If necessary, tell the client to tilt the pelvis in the posterior direction, flattening their lumbar curve, to make the *spine* more neutral. For some, the pelvis needs to be slightly posterior for the spine to feel neutral and comfortable in the supine position. It is essential that the client feel comfortable when performing supine exercises, so if necessary, tuck them under a little. This is now *their Neutral* when lying down.

SUPPORTED NEUTRAL

Neutral Spine can be supported by placing a folded up towel, deflated small ball, or sticky mat underneath any portion of the spine that is unable to make contact with the mat. This is particularly good for people with anterior pelvic tilt or lordosis (who will need a folded up towel or sticky mat under their lumbar spine so that they can feel the contact on their lumbar spines- it's like bringing the mat up to them), and also for the opposite picture; you may place a support under the lumbar spine of someone who has

a posterior pelvic tile to encourage more curvature in the lower back. Also people with too much cervical curve or forward head may need support under their head to allow the neck to lengthen as will people with. Kyphosis (these two issues often come together).

Supine Pilates stabilization exercises should never be performed with the spine unsupported (with too much extension), so make adjustments with each client individually so that they understand their Neutral Spine. Giving your client a proprioceptive tool under their back will help them to feel their abdominals engaging more and they will love you for it!

NEUTRAL SPINE VS. FLAT BACK

Many people from the New York school teach people to "tuck under" or flatten the curve of their lower back when doing Pilates exercises. In my method, I use Neutral Spine when it is safe and effective, and Flat Back when applicable.

My general rule of thumb is to use Neutral only when doing exercise that are "closed chain," meaning the legs are either on the floor *(Upper Abdominal Curl)*, or when using Pilates equipment, supported by a bar or straps *(Footwork, Leg Series)*. Pilates Mat exercises are mostly "open chain," with the legs in the air, making the spine vulnerable to destabilization. In open chain exercises, it is safer to use the Flat Back position if the client is not strong enough to stabilize in neutral (you may just choose to not give open chain exercises in this case and work on gaining stability in the neutral position first). In the Flat Back position, the Core-Tet (page 26) is slightly altered since now the multifidus muscle will be on stretch. Clients who have posterior pelvic tilt and/or very strong abdominals may experiment with bringing their pelvis more into a Neutral in open chain exercises. When on the equipment however, many exercises are closed chain, and it is an excellent opportunity to train your clients in Neutral Spine—working with the natural curves safely and effectively.

THE FOUR NEUTRALS

SUPINE NEUTRAL

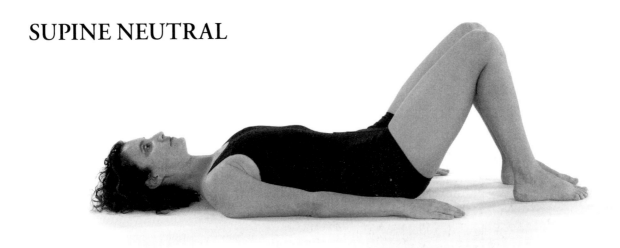

Supine Neutral is described on the previous page.

PRONE NEUTRAL

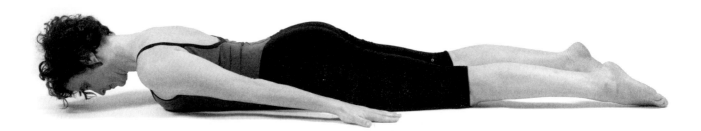

Prone Neutral is a fantastic way to find neutral spine, and can be a great way to strengthen the cervical and thoracic extensors without actually moving the spine into extension. Particularly good for people with tight lower backs who can't move their thoracic spine into extension without destabilizing their lumbar spines, and for people with stenosis, where spinal extension is painful and not recommended.

Lie on the mat face down, with legs hips distance apart in parallel. Try to find all your curves; pubic bone and hip bones on the mat, lumbar in slight extension, thoracic in slight flexion, cervical in slight extension. Then lift your head slightly, looking down to the mat, maintaining the neutral curve of the neck, and hold the head so that it is in line with the rest of the spine. Think of lengthening long in each direction, imagining the muscles that "hug" your spine pulling the spine long in both directions, through the back of the crown on your head in one direction and through your tailbone in the opposite direction. You can simply hold this position for several seconds as an exercise in and of itself, but Prone neutral is also great set up all Swans (spinal extension), and any prone exercise on the mat or equipment (Long Box on Reformer; Pulling Ropes, "T", Triceps, etc.).

SIDE-LYING NEUTRAL

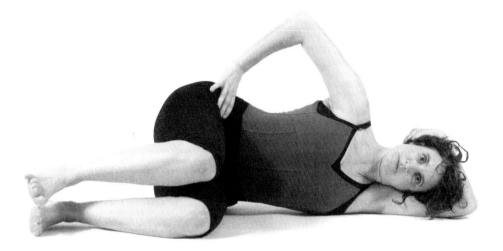

When performing side-lying exercises, make sure that the spine is in a neutral position, with head, shoulders and hips on the same line and the lower waist lifted off the mat to keep hips square. When side lying on the Arc, the lower waist is lifted, naturally creating a side lying neutral effortlessly.

QUADRUPED NEUTRAL

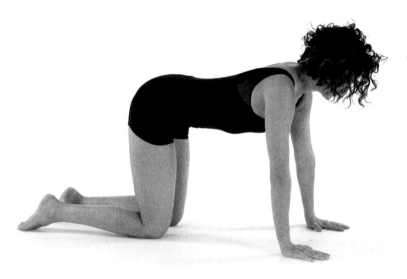

Start on your hands and knees in Neutral Spine. Perform the exercise as indicated, engaging your deep abdominals and pelvic floor without altering your bony structure (do not deviate from Neutral Spine). This is great for people who are not yet in touch with their abdominals, because lying on their back and pulling their belly in towards their spine may not feel like much at first. They may have an easier time creating a deep engagement if they have to pull their abdominals in against gravity, thus this variation.

DEMYSTIFYING THE CORE

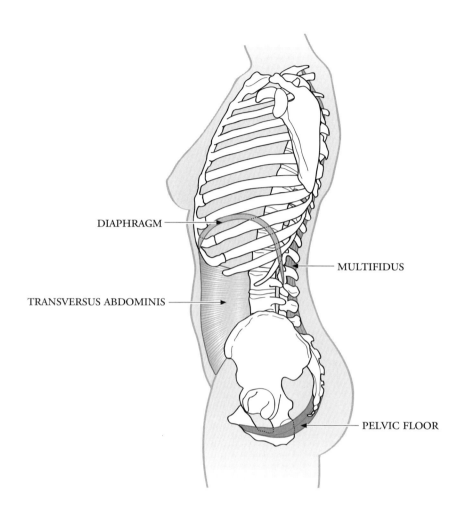

DIAPHRAGM

MULTIFIDUS

TRANSVERSUS ABDOMINIS

PELVIC FLOOR

THE "CORE-TET"

In Neutral Spine, there are four muscles that support the spine: Transversus Abdominis, Multfidus, Pelvic floor, and Diaphragm. My mentor, Doris Pasteleur-Hall, coined this phrase, the quartet and I changed to "Core-Tet."

MULTIFIDUS: THE NEW POWERHOUSE

In the world of sports medicine research, the multifidus muscle is now all the rage. Formerly thought to be relatively unimportant muscle based on its fairly small size, recent research shows that it's actually the strongest muscle in the back because of its unique structure. The Multifidus has short fibers arranged within rods which are stiffer than any other in the

body, serving a critical function as a stabilizer of the lumbar spine.

The very thin multifidus is deep in the spine, spans three joint segments, and works to stabilize the joints at each segmental level. The multifidus lies deep to the spinal erectors, transverse abdominis, and internal and external obliques.

The lumbar vertebrae carry the most body weight and are subject to the most force and stress along the spine. The multifidus muscle keeps us vertical and takes pressure off the discs.

Common wisdom in rehabilitation circles now is that injury to the spine (including surgery to treat spinal disorders) may disrupt the multifidus, decreasing spinal stability and increasing lower back pain.

THE TRANSVERSUS ABDOMINIS

The Transversus Abdominis is the deepest abdominal muscle which functions to hold the viscera in and compress the abdominal wall. Its fibers run transversely, holding the belly in like a drawstring that runs all the way around the back and attaches to lumbar fascia. And because the transversus abdominis runs transversely, it has little to no effect in flexing the spine. It is mainly a stabilizer, not a mover. And that's why it's so important for core stability, and that is also why we find the Core when the spine is in neutral. For when the spine is in flexion, as in "flat back" or posterior pelvic tilt, the other 3 abdominal muscles are now contributing to the movement, and we are no longer practicing stability in the position that your spine should live in during daily life activities. It's not wrong to do "flat back" exercises, but it turns on the superficial abdominal muscles as well as putting the multifidus muscle on stretch.

THE PELVIC FLOOR

The Pelvic Floor holds up and tones the genitals and anus and keeps other organs from bearing down and prolapsing, and it also supports the bottom of the core by lifting up from below. Some say the Pelvic Floor interdigitates with the transversus abdominis and the multifidus. To engage the Pelvic Floor, draw the two sides of your pubic bone in front closer to the two sides of your tailbone in back, forming a "hammock" lifting up from the center. Women who have been pregnant normally are advised to practice Kegel exercises to prepare for birth, and post-partum to strengthen and regain pelvic floor tone. For men, think of pulling up your family jewels. When the pelvic floor engages, one should feel a deeper engagement of the transversus and multifidus.

THE DIAPHRAGM

The Diaphragm is the major muscle of breathing but it also acts as the "top" of the Core. When you inhale, the Diaphragm contracts and dips downward, allowing air to enter the thoracic cavity. I usually have people engage their Core-Tet on the exhale, as the diaphragm eccentrically contracts and draws up, you can think of drawing the pelvic floor up with it, as if they are two parachutes connected by a string in the middle. As the diaphragm floats up, it pulls up the pelvic floor, which in turn helps to draw the belly in and lift the lumbar spine closer to the center of the body.

FINDING YOUR CORE-TET

The first step to find your "Core-Tet" is finding your neutral spine with its 3 main curves: lumbar, thoracic, and cervical. When pelvis and spine are in a neutral position, the lumbar spine has a convex curve and should be in slight extension, the thoracic spine has a concave curve and should be in slight flexion and the cervical spine has a convex curve and should be in slight extension.

You can find your Core-Tet in any position that you find neutral spine, but most commonly in the Pilates world we try to find the Core in Supine Neutral, Prone Neutral, All Fours Neutral and Side Lying Neutral. Once you've mastered finding the Core-Tet in these positions, then you can engage your core when you sit, stand and walk (which is the ultimate goal).

When the core is engaged in neutral position, we think of drawing the abdominals in toward the spine like a girdle with hooks in the back that wraps around the waist and cinches together at the spine, drawing the abdominal wall inward. Meanwhile, the lumbar spine should be in a slightly extended position when in neutral, so that the multifidus muscles that run between the vertebrae and up the spine are also engaged and "lifted." These muscles "hug" the spine like corn hugging a dog. If you think of the spine like a tall thin flexible tower that needs support, the transversus abdominis and the multifidus are like guy wires on either side supporting and stabilizing the tower against the forces pulling it in different directions.

When you find your Core-Tet you should feel a sandwich of support on the front and back of your lumbar spine as well as a feeling of lifting from the base of your pelvis up to your sternum.

THE FOUR LAYERS OF ABDOMINALS

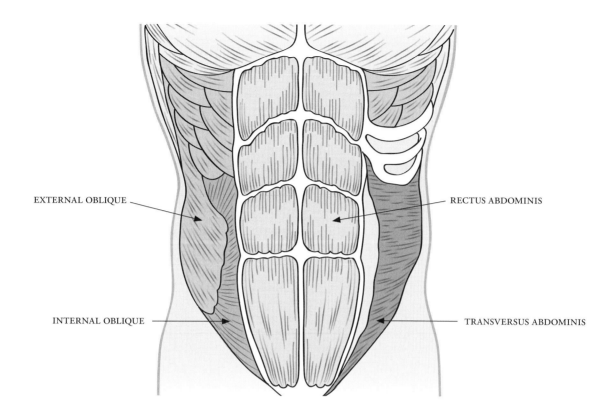

EXTERNAL OBLIQUE

RECTUS ABDOMINIS

INTERNAL OBLIQUE

TRANSVERSUS ABDOMINIS

There are four layers of abdominals; the deepest layer is the **Transversus Abdominis** whose fibers run transversely, all the way around the waist and attach to the fascia of the back. The Transversus, when contracted, acts like a drawstring on a pair of sweat pants, decreasing the circumference of the waist, and compressing the abdomen. It functions to hold your viscera in and acts like a girdle of support for your spine.

The next two layers are your **Internal** and **External Obliques** which, when contracted also compress the abdomen, and working synergistically, allow your spine to side bend, rotate and twist.

And last but not least, there's the **Rectus Abdominis**, the "workaholic" of the abdominals—whose main function is flexion of the trunk. One could perform a trunk curl simply by using the Rectus Abdominis which would "pooch" one's belly out. Or one could do a Pilates *Upper Abdominal Curl* engaging the "deep three"

(Transversus, Internal and External Obliques) in addition to the rectus abdominis, by scooping the belly in and trying to maintain this scoop while curling the trunk.

When one keeps the scoop during a trunk curl, the "deep three" come into play, which help support the spine and prevent injury. This would be the Pilates way.

The Rectus Abdominis gets a bad rap in much of the Pilates world, and I would like to hail some of the virtues of this underrated little six pack. Without the Rectus Abdominis, we could not come up into a full trunk curl, nor hold our heads up in exercises like the *Hundred*. In addition, the Rectus Abdominis, which runs from the pubic bone to sternum, has the most direct line of pull to correct anterior pelvic tilt and lordosis. So, it's not that we want to never use the Rectus Abdominis, it's just that we want to use it in moderation, bringing in the other three abdominals to synergistically assist the rectus in spinal flexion and stabilization exercises.

SPINAL FLEXION: WHAT YOU NEED TO KNOW

Spinal Flexion is one of the most common movements done in the Pilates Method.

FUNCTIONS

• Strengthens the abdominals, when supine

• Stretches the extensor muscles of the back

• Great for people with anterior pelvic tilt and lordosis (particularly lumbar flexion exercises)

GENERAL OBSTACLES

Like any movement, tightness in the oppositional muscle group will inhibit Range of Motion in the working muscle. With spinal flexion, the main movers are the abdominals and the opposing muscle groups are the back extensors. So if the back extensors are tight, in any portion of the spine, then it will be difficult to flex that part of the back.

For example, if someone has trouble coming up into an *Upper Abdominal Curl*, generally that points to a tightness in the neck and upper back. If someone has trouble imprinting their lower back onto the mat during a *Roll Down* or rolling exercise, then they probably have a tight lower back.

UNIVERSAL CONTRAINDICATIONS

Because flexing the spine puts pressure and load onto the anterior structures of the spine; i.e. the intervertebral discs and bodies of the vertebrae, then any weakness or dysfunction of the anterior structures will make that person vulnerable to injury when flexing the spine. The more loaded the flexion, the more damaging. Please refer to the Loaded Flexion Continuum Chart (opposite page) for an overview of Pilates exercises and their concomitant load.

• DISC DYSFUNCTION

The intervertebral discs live in between the vertebral bodies of the spine and function as shock absorbers and cushioners for the huge amount of compression that loads the back every day. Most disc injuries are due to daily life activities that load the spine in flexion and ultimately weaken, herniate, or "slip" one or more discs. The following are the most common disc dysfunctions:

• **Degeneration:** Degeneration happens to all of us as we age, causing the disc to flatten due to the loss of its inner fluids. With too much degeneration, the cushioning action of the discs is lessened and inflammation and micro movements of the vertebral bodies that sandwich the discs can cause chronic pain.

• **Herniation:** A herniated disc is caused by the rupture of the cartilaginous outer layer which allows the inner fluid to escape into the spaces near the nerve roots along the spine—ouch!

• **Subluxation:** A disc can simply "slip" out of its normal position and move anteriorly onto the nerve roots (double ouch!)—this is called subluxation.

In all these cases of disc dysfunction, loaded flexion would most likely be contraindicated and would greatly exacerbate any symptoms. Some disc problems are exacerbated by extension, but the majority can be relieved by extension.

• OSTEOPOROSIS

Osteoporosis is defined as a decrease in bone mass and bone density with an increased risk and/or incidence of fracture. Women over 50 should get checked to make sure they aren't suffering from osteoporosis or osteopenia (a less severe version). Flexion exercises are universally contraindicated for these conditions because it loads the vertebral bodies which are weakened and vulnerable to breakage. Instead, do exercises where the spine is in neutral or extension.

LOADED SPINAL FLEXION CONTINUUM

| LEAST LOADED | SEMI LOADED | VERY LOADED! |

SPINAL EXTENSION: WHAT YOU NEED TO KNOW

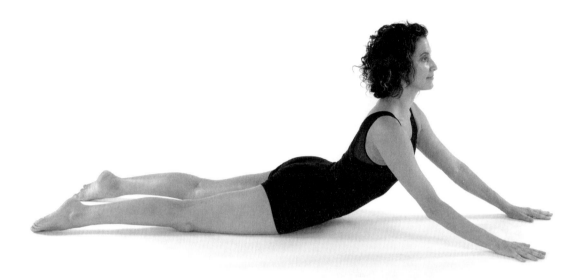

Back extension exercises when performed prone (on your belly), actively use your spinal extensors. In many Pilates Mat exercises, spinal extension originates from the head and neck and sequences through the spine to the upper back and finally the lower back.

FUNCTIONS

• Strengthens the spine and neck extensors when prone

• Stretches the front body; namely the abdominals and chest

• Great for people with posterior pelvic tilt, who generally present with lengthened lumbar extensors and tight abdominals. For these people, it is not as essential to initiate full back extension with the hip extensors since they are already living in a relatively "tucked" position

• Great for people with kyphosis (particularly upper back extension exercises)

CAUTION

Be mindful when training people with lordosis and anterior pelvic tilt since those individuals will have short/tight lumbar extensors and hip flexors along with weak/lengthened abdominals and hip extensors (glutes and hamstrings). They should only do the *Cygnet* (baby *Swan*), lifting only their head, neck, and upper back, keeping their lower back stable, using the Abdominal Scoop and hip extensors (glutes and hamstrings) to stabilize the pelvis. This should feel like a butt and hamstring exercise for these people, not a lower back exercise.

UNIVERSAL CONTRAINDICATIONS

Because extending the spine puts pressure and load onto the posterior structures of the spine; i.e. the spinal canal and the facet joints, then any weakness or dysfunction of the posterior structures will make that person vulnerable to injury when extending the spine. The more loaded the extension, the more damaging.

• STENOSIS

Spinal stenosis is the narrowing of the lumbar spinal canal, an arthritic process, which happens as a normal part of aging. People with this problem will experience minor to severe nerve impingement.

• FACET JOINT PROBLEMS

Facet joints are in almost constant motion with the spine and simply wear out and/or degenerate in people as they age. When facet joints become worn there may be a reaction of the bone of the joint underneath producing bone spurs and an enlargement of the joints (osteoarthritis). This condition may also be referred to as "facet joint disease" or "facet joint syndrome" and can be quite painful for people when they move their spine. In both the case of stenosis and facet joint problems, extension will exacerbate symptoms and flexion and/or Neutral Spine may alleviate them.

• OSTEOPOROSIS AND STENOSIS

Flexion of the spine is contraindicated for people who have osteoporosis and extension of the spine is contraindicated for people with stenosis...what do you do with people who have both osteoporosis and stenosis? Three words: Neutral, Neutral and Neutral.

DISC DYSFUNCTION

Be careful doing any extreme spinal movements with clients who are suffering from disc dysfunction. However, gentle and passive extension of the spine can be indicated for people suffering from vertebral disc dysfunction (herniated, bulging or subluxated disc) because it opens the space between the vertebral bodies anteriorly and allows the disc to return to its proper space, away from the spinal nerve roots which, when impinged, cause pain. There is no reason to do thoracic flexion.

KYPHOSIS

Passive extension is the best way to train a client with Kyphosis. Have the client lie back over a Pilates Arc, small ball, or rolled up blanket underneath their shoulder blades. From this position also do eccentric abdominal curls, starting in extension and stopping at neutral. There is no reason to into thoracic flexion with these clients. Eccentric abdominal curls are also excellent for people with osteoporosis.

THE ROLE OF HIP EXTENSORS

Back Extension and Hip Extension flow together since the base of the spine (sacrum) is shared and continuous with the hips and pelvis. Full back extension (think: *High Swan*), cannot be fully achieved without hip extension.

Spinal Extension should be initiated by hip extensors and abdominals to protect the lower back from hyperextension and to allow full spinal extension. This means starting every time with scooping the belly in and tucking your pelvis under with your glutes and hamstrings.

People with weakness in their hip extensors (glutes and hamstrings) will not be able to do full back extension in a prone position because the pelvis cannot stabilize on the mat and the spine will not be able to fully lift off the mat. This issue is often coupled with/caused by tight hip flexors.

THE ROLE OF ABDOMINALS

Scooping the abdominals in toward the spine while attempting Spinal Extension will help to distribute the extension throughout the spine. When abdominals are not engaged, most of the back extension will occur at L2–3.

Thus, it is essential when doing prone full back extension exercises to initiate the movement with both the abdominals and hip extensors. I always cue "scoop your belly in toward your spine, squeeze your glutes and tuck your pelvis under, and then rise up into back extension."

ASSISTING PEOPLE

When teaching prone back extension exercises to folks with weak abdominals, glutes and hamstrings, I recommend assisting them to prevent compression in their lumbar spines. Hold their calves down (or you can strap their legs down if you have access to a Cadilllac) so they can stabilize their pelvis and activate their glutes and hamstrings. This will enable them to rise all the way up into a full *Swan*. Try it—you'll see them rise like a phoenix from the ashes.

BREAKING DOWN THE FULL TRUNK CURL

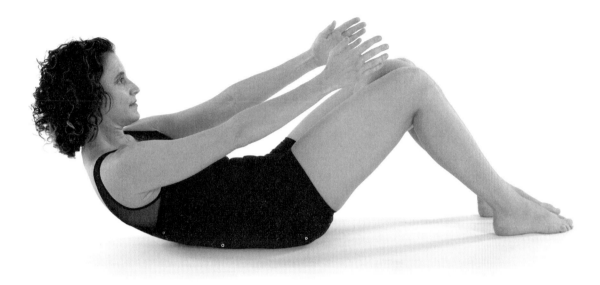

Ellie is rolling up; transitioning from the Abdominal Phase into the Hip Flexion phase.

EXERCISES

- Roll Down
- Roll Up
- Neck Pull
- Teasers
- Balance Point*

A FULL TRUNK CURL HAS TWO PHASES:

1) Abdominal Phase: this is the first stage of a sit up when starting supine, and brings a person up to the point where the spine can no longer flex, normally 40 degrees from the floor. The Abdominal Curl is an example of an exercise which works the spine only in the Abdominal Phase.

2) Hip Flexion Phase: this completes the sit up, and is mainly performed by the psoas muscle. The goal of a Pilates Roll Down (or Roll Up for that matter) is to maximize the abdominal phase of a full sit up. This is accomplished by imprinting the lower back into the mat as one articulates down and up.

When the lower abdominals are weak and hip flexors are strong, (as seen in people with anterior pelvic tilt

and lordosis), the lower back will skip the imprinting phase of the movement, and stay relatively extended instead of fully flexed and pressed into the mat. This is especially noticeable in the rolling up direction—if a person has weak lower abdominals you will see a shortened abdominal phase (instead of imprinting their lower back onto the mat to smoothly articulate up, there will be a slight "heaving" up to the sit up position as they lever up from their hip flexors). In this case the lower back will straighten and lift off the mat instead of imprinting.

When the psoas activates to pull one up to a sitting position, it wants to extend the lower back—that is why it is essential to teach these exercises slowly and carefully (and giving assisted resistance when necessary) so they don't just keep shortening and strengthening the psoas without addressing the weak area: the lower abs! This is a very common problem and must be fixed!

* **Balance Point.** Although a full trunk curl exercise, since the legs are being supported by the arms, and the legs are pressing into the arms, the hip flexion phase becomes a hip extension phase instead, thereby removing the hip flexors from the equation. This is why we love it so much, especially for folks with overactive hip flexors and under-utilized abdominals.

HOW TO CREATE AN HOUR-LONG SESSION

Think of the repertoire as your palette, from which you, the Pilates artist, should pick and choose based on your knowledge of what you or your client needs.

When planning a Pilates class make sure that you:

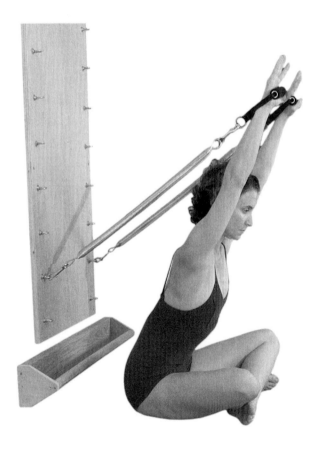

1. WORK ALL PARTS OF THE BODY

Spine: We can break down spinal exercises into **stabilization** and **articulation**. It is important to do both kinds of core strengthening, but equally important to notice if your client needs more of one than the other. For instance, if you are training a very stiff, tight client whose spine barely moves in any direction, then articulation exercises will be preferable to stabilization exercises. And conversely, if you have a noodle-y client who is hyper-mobile and can't keep her trunk still to save her life, then stabilization would make more sense for her.

*Rehabilitation Note: When working with clients who have spinal injuries, especially disc dysfunction, stabilization is the preferred core strengthening technique. Spinal flexion or extension (or any extreme spinal movement) may exacerbate certain back injuries.

Spinal Stabilization:
Exercises: *Hundred, Coordination, Plank, Control Front,* and *Flat Back* versions of most exercises.

Spinal Articulation:
Exercises: *Rolling Like a Ball, Roll Downs, Teasers,* and *Round Back* versions of most exercises

Lower Body:
Exercises: *all Leg Springs exercises, Squats,* and *Jumping*

Upper Body:
Exercises: *all Arm Springs exercises, Tricep* and *Lat Presses*

Total Body: Some exercises on the Springboard work your whole body in resistance, and these are good to include in every workout.
Exercises: *Arabesque, Jumping, Squat with Arm Pulls, all Lunging exercises,* and *all Kneeling exercises*

2. MOVE THE SPINE IN ALL DIRECTIONS

Flexion: Generally we start the workout with flexion exercises because it fires up our abdominals and warms up the spine.
Exercises: *Hundred, Hip Ups, Rolling Like a Ball, Roll Down Round Back, Teaser*

Extension: After doing a series of flexion exercises, make sure to do spinal extension exercises to balance the spine.
Exercises: *Roll Back Arch Back, Swan,* and *3-Way Pec Stretch*

Side Bending or Lateral Flexion: Side bending stretches out the abdominal obliques and quadratus lumborum and can help lateral imbalances like scoliosis.
Exercises: *Side Roll Ups* and *Painting Under the Stairs*

Twisting: Twisting is healthy for the spine, but it is not indicated for disc dysfunction.
Exercises: *Twist Round Back* and *Twist Flat Back*

3. LET THE SESSION FLOW

Choose an exercise order that makes sense for flow so that you don't have to change the springs with each exercise and so your client is not getting up and off the machine every minute.

Think of the repertoire as your palette, from which you, the Pilates artist, should pick and choose based on your knowledge of what you or your client needs.

See the Ellie Herman Workout DVD for an example of a Springboard workout flow.

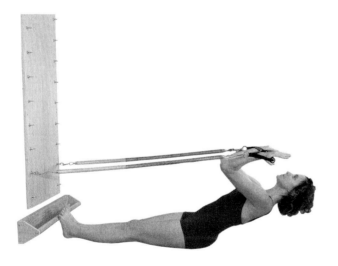

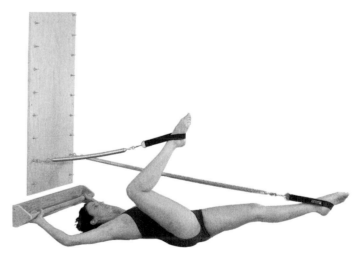

HOW TO USE THIS MANUAL

The manual has what I consider to be a complete repertoire of Pilates Arc & Barrel Exercises; some are classic Pilates, while others are invented by myself or other trainers over the years.

THE LEVELS
We have broken down the levels into:
• **Beginning**
• **Intermediate**
• **Advanced**
• **Super Advanced**

THE SERIES
In the Pilates Method, the Reformer and the Mat are taught as series, meaning each level has a specific order and flow. (Exercises on the Cadillac, Chair, and Barrel are not generally taught in a series; they are discrete and can be added in to a workout to address specific issues you or your client may have.)

When teaching a client in a one-hour time frame, you will have to use your best judgment when deciding what is essential for that client. You will may not be able to do all the exercises in a given level in one hour. (Even the beginning series can be quite long!) The series is really a way to organize the exercises, giving you a framework and an order.

Beginning Series: Start at the beginning of the manual and go in order, doing all of the beginning exercises.

Intermediate Series: Start at the beginning of the manual and do the essential beginning and all the intermediate exercises in order. Any exercise that has a beginning version and an intermediate version, replace with the more advanced version and omit the easier one.

Advanced and Super Advanced Series: Start at the beginning of the manual and do all the beginning and intermediate exercises and selected advanced and super advanced exercises in order. For any exercise that has both an intermediate and an advanced version, do the more advanced version and omit the easier one.

Remember, the levels of the exercises are meant to help you learn the Pilates Method in a natural progression for your body. Most importantly, the levels are meant to help you not hurt yourself. The intermediate and advanced exercises require a fair amount of core strength to perform properly. You could injure yourself or your client if you try to push beyond the appropriate level.

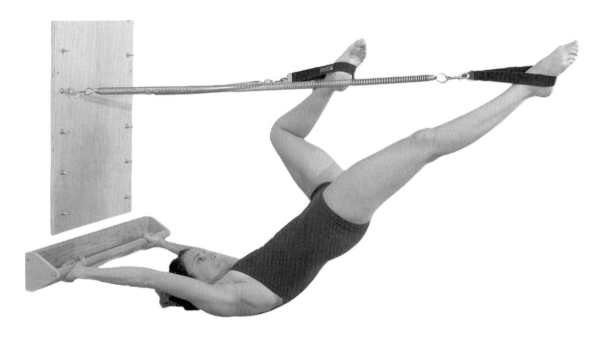

OTHER HELPFUL THINGS

Please read the Cues and Obstacles sections for each exercise carefully to make sure you understand the correct form.

As a teacher, "do no harm" is your most important mantra! So read the **contraindications** carefully to make sure you're not hurting yourself or anyone else.

Specific modifications are outlined in each exercise if there are any. They are meant to help you advance at your own pace. If you or your client feel strain in your low back or neck at anytime, or if the exercise is just too difficult, please do not continue with the movement; look for modifications instead.

GENERAL MODIFICATIONS

When learning new exercises it is common for certain aches and pains to develop. The following are a few common problems that people face when they are still in the process of gaining strength and stability. Please read through this section even if you don't have any of these problems yet. The point is to prevent potential overuse or strain of your muscles and tissues.

How to modify to protect the low back:
In general, if you suffer from low back pain, you need to know a few tips to keep you from further contributing to your problems. Always modify any exercise that requires you to support your legs out in front of you while keeping your belly scooped or your back flat on the mat. Experiment with the following modifications:

• Bend your knees if the exercise requires straight legs.

• Keep your legs high enough so that you can absolutely maintain a scooped belly and a flat back on the mat.

• Stop if you feel back strain.

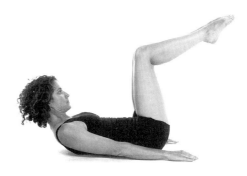

PROTECT YOUR LOW BACK: BEGINNING

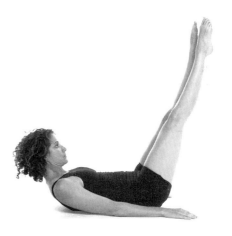

PROTECT YOUR LOW BACK: INTERMEDIATE

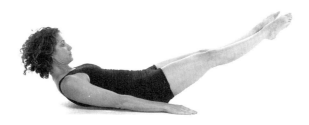

PROTECT YOUR LOW BACK: ADVANCED

How to avoid wrist compression when up on your arms:

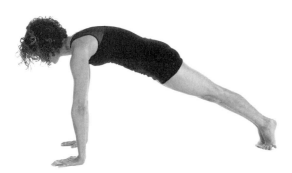

PROTECT YOUR WRISTS: CORRECT—LIFT UP FROM THE WRISTS AND SHOULDERS AND SOFTEN THE ELBOWS

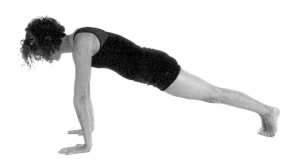

PROTECT YOUR WRISTS: INCORRECT—AVOID DROPPING INTO YOUR WRISTS, ELBOWS, AND SHOULDERS

- Keep your shoulders properly aligned. Think of rolling the shoulder blades down away from the ears so you are supporting your body weight from the back muscles.

- Think of pressing away from the mat with your back strength.

- Don't let your weight bear down into the wrist; instead, press away from gravity.

- Don't hyperextend your elbows: keep the inner elbow creases facing each other.

How to do a rolling exercise: Never onto your neck!

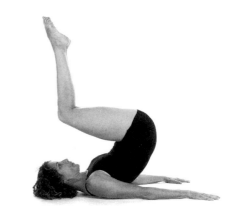

CORRECT NECK PLACEMENT: BALANCE BETWEEN YOUR SHOULDER BLADES ON YOUR "THORACIC SHELF"

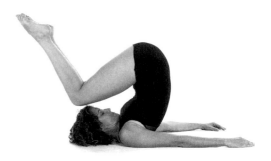

INCORRECT NECK PLACEMENT: DON'T ROLL ONTO YOUR NECK

There are several exercises on the Mat that require you to roll onto your upper back (Rolling Like a Ball, Roll Over, etc.).

- Do not roll onto your neck; instead, stop and balance between your shoulder blades.

- Use control when rolling back. Don't roll back so fast that you can't control your momentum.

- Scoop your abdominals in to help stop yourself from rolling back too far.

EXERCISES

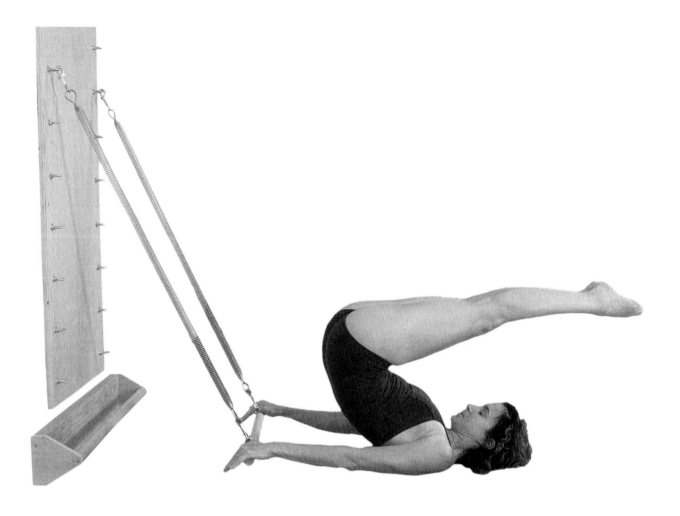

Notes on spring resistance for all exercises:

• When doing exercises down on the floor, raising the springs will increase resistance

• When doing exercises standing or lunging, the resistance can be increased <u>or</u> decreased by raising the springs—
  always look at the angle of the springs. When the spring is straight, it has the least resistance; when it is at an
  angle, it has the most resistance.

If you have a new Springboard (that goes up to 11), please make sure to adjust the springs accordingly, raising them
up 1–2 eyebolts from the settings listed.

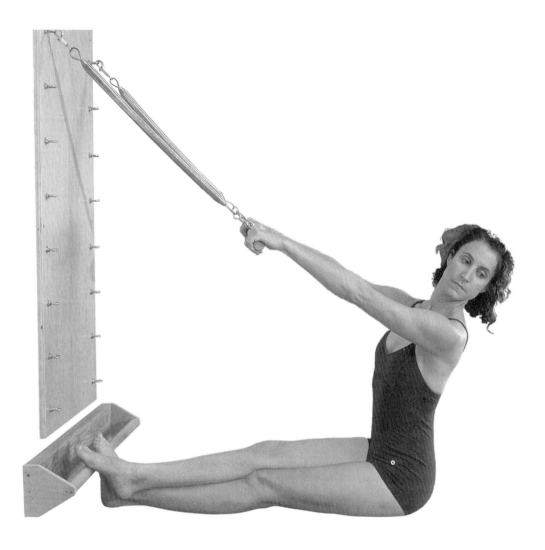

The Roll-Down Bar is classically a part of the Cadillac (or Trap Table) and consists of two yellow arm springs and a wooden dowel.

The Roll-Down Bar is the most versatile modality on the Pilates Springboard and addresses all parts of the body. I could do an hour-long full body conditioning class with just this piece of wood and a couple springs!

Many of the Roll-Down Bar exercises in this book are part of the classical Pilates repertoire, (*Roll Downs, Pilates Squat*) while others have been translated from the push-thru bar on the Cadillac (*Swan, Seated Chicken Wings*). Still others are classical Pilates exercises with a twist (*Rolling Like a Ball, Teaser, Jackknife*). And lastly there are several original exercises developed by myself or my trainers over the years which use Pilates concepts but take it a little further…(*Jumping, Arabesque, Levitated Hip Fold*).

ROLL-DOWN BAR SET UP

- 6th or 7th eyebolt from the floor
- Adjust 1–2 eyebolts higher if you have a newer Springboard that goes up to 10 or 11

FUNCTIONS & TARGET MUSCLES

- Cues the deep abdominals, especially the transversus abdominis
- Teaches pelvic stability in neutral, while legs move freely

ALIGNMENT CUES & OBSTACLES

- Keep the belly scooped, especially as the legs lower
- Keep pelvis neutral and stable while legs move

VARIATIONS & PEEL BACKS

- Try flexing your feet and touching your heels
- Keep the feet close to the floor and pulse toes down, then heels, then toes, etc.

IMAGINE...*your legs move independently from your torso.*

ELLIE SAYS...*"This is a great way to start a springboard class."*

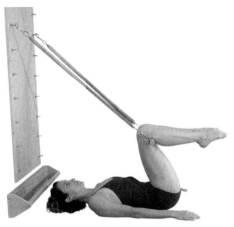

1. Starting Position — *10 times touching toes, 10 times touching heels, 10 times alternating*
Lie on your back with your head close to the Springboard and pull the roll-down bar down. Put your legs in between the springs so that the back of your knees fold, and hold onto the roll-down bar. Roll up your pants so that the bare skin is against the wood (this makes it easier to maintain the bar in place). Place your hands on your low belly to help cue the deep abs.

Inhale to prepare

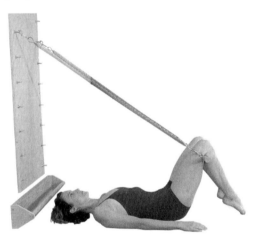

2. Exhale
Scoop your belly in and feel the low abs compress as you lower your legs, touching the toes to the floor. Inhale as you return to the starting position.

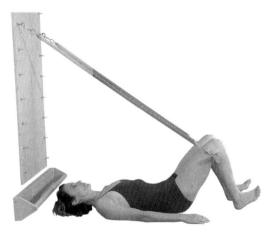

3. Breathing Continuously
Try flexing feet and alternating heels, toes, heels, toes in a percussive rhythm, keeping scoop in low belly!

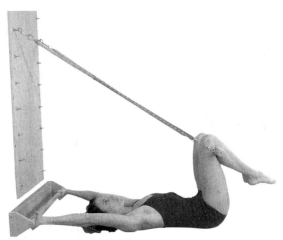

1. Starting Position — *10 repetitions*

Lie on your back with your head close to the Springboard and pull down the roll-down bar. Put your legs in between the springs so that the back of your knees fold, and hold onto the roll-down bar. Roll up your pants so that the bare skin is against the wood (this makes it easier to maintain the bar in place). Hold onto the stability bar and press yourself away as far as you can.

Inhale to prepare

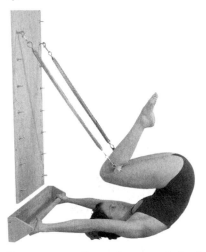

2. Exhale

Scoop your belly in as you roll your hips up off the floor. Think knees to chest first, then hips up.

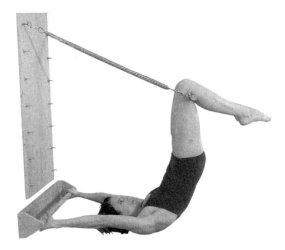

3. Inhale

Inhale to retrograde the movement, bringing your knees to your chest as you roll back down.

ROLL-DOWN BAR SET UP

- 6th or 7th eyebolt from the floor
- Adjust 1–2 eyebolts higher if you have a newer Springboard that goes up to 10 or 11

FUNCTIONS & TARGET MUSCLES

- Strengthens lower abs
- Teaches levitation

ALIGNMENT CUES & OBSTACLES

- Keep pressing your body away from the Springboard with strong, long arms
- Place your arms down by your sides if you feel tension in your neck and upper back, or bend your arms while holding the bar
- Never roll onto your neck, instead balance between your shoulder blades
- **Contraindications:** Disc dysfunction, osteoporosis, neck problems

VARIATIONS & PEEL BACKS

- **Variation:** *Half Moon*: Think of making a circle with your knees; first bring knees to your chest, then lift the hips in levitation but instead of landing on your feet, levitate a little less and land on your tailbone, still reaching your legs away from you. Reverse by levitating your hips up, reaching your knees away from you, then bring the knees up and into your chest to roll down your spine.

IMAGINE...*you are massaging your spine as you roll up and down.*

ELLIE SAYS...*"This is how to teach the hip-up on the mat for those with big butts, weak abs, or tight lower backs."*

VARIATION: Half Moon

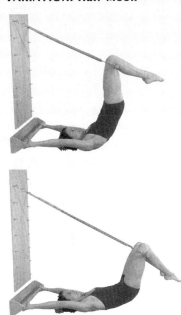

ROLL-DOWN BAR SET UP

- 6th–9th eyebolt from the floor
- Adjust 1–2 eyebolts higher if you have a newer Springboard that goes up to 10 or 11

FUNCTIONS & TARGET MUSCLES

- Strengthens lower abs
- Teaches levitation

ALIGNMENT CUES & OBSTACLES

- Keep pressing your body away from the Springboard with strong long arms
- Place your arms down by your sides if you feel tension in the neck and upper back
- Never roll onto your neck; instead balance between your shoulder blades
- **Contraindications:** Disc dysfunction, osteoporosis, neck problems

VARIATIONS & PEEL BACKS

- **Peel Backs:** *Hip Ups* and *Half Moon*

IMAGINE...*you are a parakeet on a swing.*

ELLIE SAYS...*"Watch out for your traps!"*

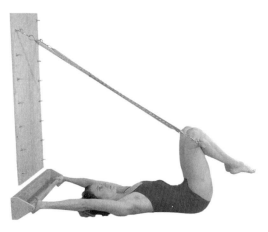

1. Starting Position — *3 repetitions and reverse*

Lie on your back with your head close to the Springboard and pull down the roll-down bar, putting your legs in between the springs so that the back of your knees fold and hold onto the roll-down bar. Roll up your pants so that the bare skin is against the wood (this makes it easier to maintain the bar in place). Hold onto the stability bar and press yourself away as far as you can. Place your feet on the mat.

Inhale to prepare

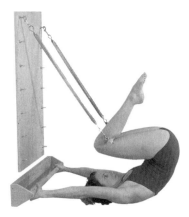

2. Exhale

Start with a *hip-up*, scooping your belly in as you lift your hips up off the floor. Think knees to chest first, then hips up.

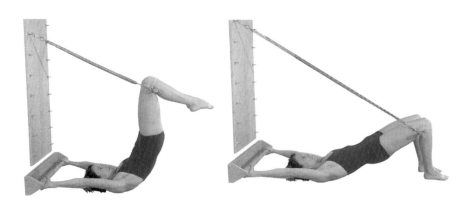

3. Inhale

Levitate your hips at the top of the *hip-up* by squeezing your glutes, and land like a cat on your feet. You should land in a bridge.

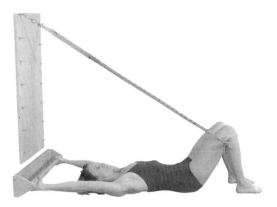

4. Exhale
Roll down one vertebra at a time, coming back to the starting position.

Repeat 3 times, then retrograde the movement as follows:

Inhale to prepare

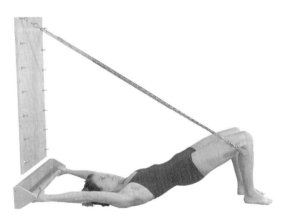

5. Exhale
Keeping your feet pressing onto the mat, coccyx curl your hips up into a bridge.

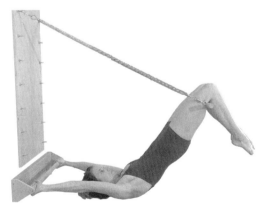

6. Inhale
Levitate your hips up to the sky by squeezing your glutes and using your feet to press off the floor.

7. Exhale
Bring your knees to your chest and roll down your spine until you return to the starting position.

Repeat 3 times.

LEVITATED HIP FOLD

ROLL-DOWN BAR SET UP

- 6th–9th eyebolt from the floor
- Use long leg springs here and attach it to the roll back bar
- Adjust 1–2 eyebolts higher if you have a newer Springboard that goes up to 10 or 11

FUNCTIONS & TARGET MUSCLES

- Strengthens lower abs
- Teaches levitation

ALIGNMENT CUES & OBSTACLES

- Keep pressing your body away from the Springboard with strong long arms
- Place your arms down by your sides if you feel tension in the neck and upper back
- Never roll onto your neck; instead balance between your shoulder blades
- **Contraindications:** Disc dysfunction, osteoporosis, neck problems

VARIATIONS & PEEL BACKS

- **Variation:** *Levitated Knee Circle*: From your last hip fold, maintaining levitation, bend your knees in toward your chest and then extend the legs to a low plank. The hips will follow as the knees circle up in and out. The hips never touch down to the floor. Do 3 circles and reverse direction.

IMAGINE...*you have run off to join the circus.*

ELLIE SAYS...*"I feel like a trapeze artist"*

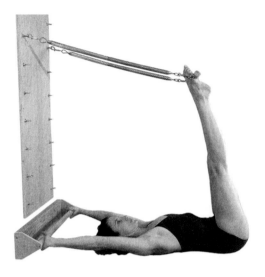

1. Starting Position — *3 repetitions and reverse*
Lie on your back with your head close to the Springboard and pull down the roll-down bar to carefully place the arches of your feet on the bar, a few inches apart, making sure you have a good purchase. Press away with your arms for support.

Inhale to prepare

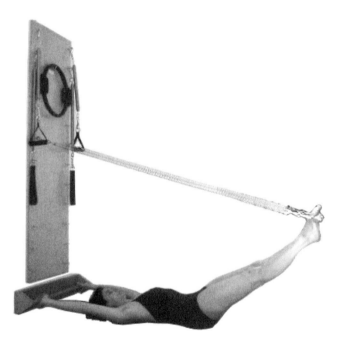

2. Exhale Down and Inhale Up
Start with 3–5 leg pulls, keeping pelvis grounded to mat, pulling the bar down to about 30 degrees from the floor.

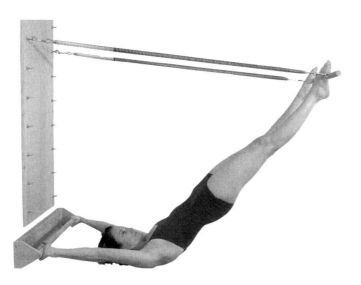

3. Inhale

At the bottom of your leg pull, levitate your hips up so that your body is in one long plank.

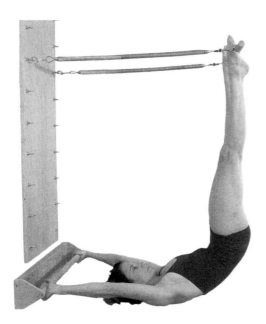

4. Exhale

Fold at the hip and roll down one vertebra at a time until your pelvis is down on the mat, returning to starting position.

VARIATION: Levitated Knee Circle

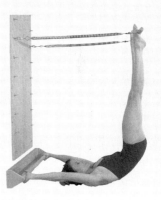

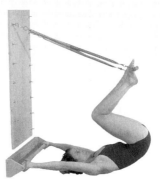

ROLL DOWN ROUND BACK

ROLL-DOWN BAR SET UP

- 6th or 7th eyebolt from the floor
- Adjust 1–2 eyebolts higher if you have a newer Springboard that goes up to 10 or 11

FUNCTIONS & TARGET MUSCLES

- Strengthens abdominals
- Stretches spinal extensors
- Teaches spinal articulation and stacking the spine, is a peel back for *Roll Downs* in mat work

ALIGNMENT CUES & OBSTACLES

- When rolling down, initiate the C-Curve with the low abdominals and lumbar spine
- Keep the oppositional energy of the "golden string" lengthening the spine as you begin your C-Curve descent
- When rolling up, resist with your belly to create the best spine stretch possible
- Do not initiate roll down by dropping the head and rounding upper back—keep middle trapezius working to stabilize shoulder girdle
- Keep elbows straight
- Keep hip flexors as soft as possible to make sure the abdominals are doing the bulk of the work
- **Contraindications:** Unstable Sacroiliac joint (can be exacerbated in seated flexion), disc problems in neck, disc dysfunction, osteoporosis

VARIATIONS & PEEL BACKS

- If the hip flexors are overworking, place pillows under client's knees for support to relax the legs and concentrate on the abdominals
- For more challenge, straighten the legs. This is not recommended for clients with tight backs, because straightening the legs makes it difficult to articulate the spine.

IMAGINE...you are doing a coccyx curl from the sitting position to initiate the roll back.

ELLIE SAYS..."This is a classic Pilates exercise to get the spine moving."

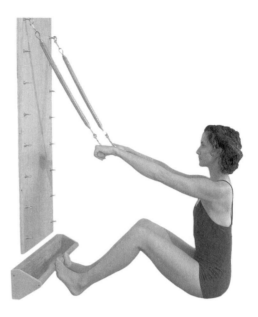

1. Starting Position — *3 repetitions*
Sit facing Springboard, holding onto roll-down bar with hands outside of the springs, thumbs with fingers. Knees are bent with feet flexed, heels on the mat and the balls of the feet pressing into the foot bar.

Inhale to prepare and imagine a "golden string" lifting you up from the top of your head

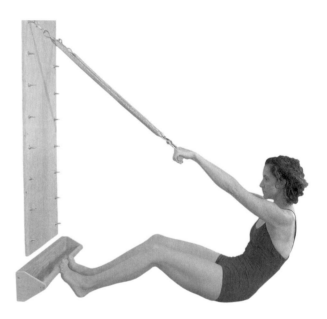

2. Exhale
Pull your abdominals toward your spine to round the lumbar, and begin to roll down through the spine, one vertebra at a time. Move sequentially through tailbone, sacrum, then lumbar spine. Pause when your lumbar spine is imprinted onto the mat.

3. Inhale
Maintain position of torso.

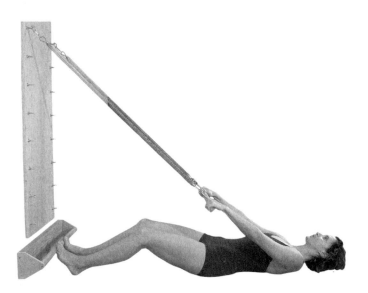

4. Exhale
Continue to roll down through spine until you are lying flat on the mat. Release shoulders into mat.

5. Inhale

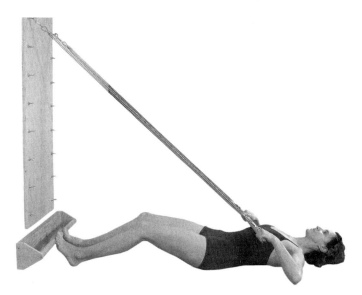

ADVANCED VARIATION:
Legs Straight

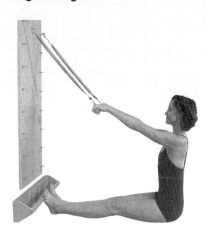

6. Exhale
Pull the roll-down bar to your sternum, keeping your elbows wide and your shoulders open and away from the ears.

7. Inhale
Straighten arms and repeat arm pulls 3 times.

8. Exhale
Lengthen the back of your neck, then lift head to "squeeze a tangerine" under your chin and begin to roll up sequentially through spine, allowing the humerus to roll forward to allow thoracic rounding. Come onto sits bones maintaining entire spine C-Curve.

9. Inhale
Stack up from the base of the spine, bringing head into alignment last.

10. Exhale
Drop the shoulders down the back.

ROLL-DOWN BAR SET UP

- 6th or 7th eyebolt from the floor
- Adjust 1–2 eyebolts higher if you have a newer Springboard that goes up to 10 or 11

FUNCTIONS & TARGET MUSCLES

- Teaches spinal stabilization, especially head and neck alignment
- Strengthens the abdominals and hip flexors
- Works spinal extensors

ALIGNMENT CUES & OBSTACLES

- Keep eyes focused in front of you—don't allow your head to lead you back
- Only your head or hair will touch the mat behind you...and don't dally back there

VARIATIONS & PEEL BACKS

- **Modification:** If client is too weak or unstable, decrease ROM

IMAGINE...you are free-falling backward into a trusted friend's arms.

ELLIE SAYS..."Think 'hot potato' and when your head hits the mat, rebound back to sitting."

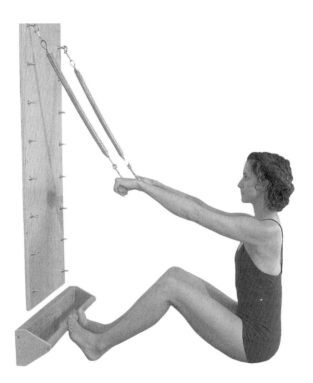

1. Starting Position — *5 repetitions*
Sit facing Springboard and hold roll-down bar with hands outside of springs, thumbs with fingers. Knees are bent with feet flexed, heels on the mat and the balls of the feet pressing into foot bar.

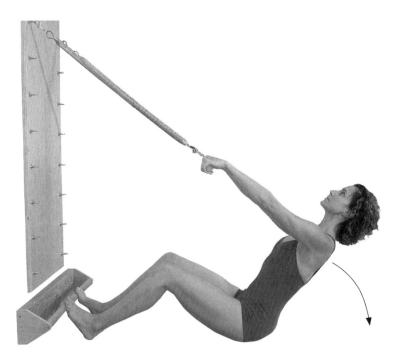

2. Inhale
Hinge back, keeping the chest lifted and the head and neck stable. Do not round lumbar spine. Go down until your hair touches the mat.

3. Exhale
Rebound back to sitting, maintaining a lifted chest, accenting the "up" motion.

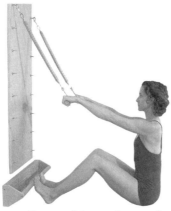

1. Starting Position — *2 repetitions alternating*

Sit facing Springboard and hold roll-down bar with hands outside of the springs, thumbs with fingers. Knees are bent with feet flexed, heels on the mat and the balls of the feet pressing into the foot bar.

Inhale to prepare and sit tall imagining a "golden string" at the top and back of your head lengthening your spine

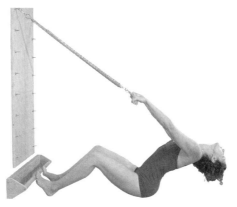

2. Exhale

Lift the chest and arch the back, releasing the head backward until the top of your head touches the mat.

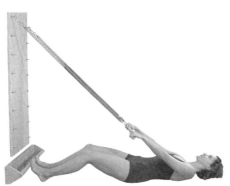

Step 3

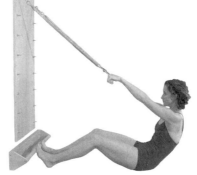

Step 4

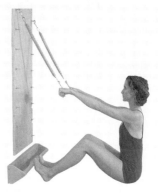

Step 5

3. Inhale

Slide the back of the neck along the mat until you are lying back on the mat with neck in neutral.

4. Exhale

Squeeze a tangerine under your chin to roll up, one vertebra at a time.

5. Inhale

Stack up the spine. Exhale. Drop the shoulders down the back.

Reverse: Start with a *Round Back Roll Down*, coming down to lying flat. Then lift the chest to rise back up as if a string is attached to your sternum, lifting you up, then stack up the spine to finish.

ROLL-DOWN BAR SET UP

- 6th or 7th eyebolt from the floor
- Adjust 1–2 eyebolts higher if you have a newer Springboard that goes up to 10 or 11

FUNCTIONS & TARGET MUSCLES

- Stretches the chest and front of the neck
- Releases the head and neck in extension
- Works abdominals and back extensors

ALIGNMENT CUES & OBSTACLES

- Avoid straining neck by allowing the arching movement to flow
- Your head must be fully released back—not half-mast
- Even though you are arching back, don't pop your ribs—use your abdominals, too
- Keep low and mid trapezius engaged to keep shoulders away from the ears while extending the spine
- **Contraindications:** Neck injuries, Stenosis

VARIATIONS & PEEL BACKS

- **Peel Back:** *Round Back Roll Down*

IMAGINE...you have a string pulling you up from your sternum as you make your way back to sitting.

ELLIE SAYS..."This exercise is not right for everyone...teach it judiciously."

ROLL-DOWN BAR SET UP

- 6th or 7th eyebolt from the floor
- Adjust 1–2 eyebolts higher if you have a newer Springboard that goes up to 10 or 11

FUNCTIONS & TARGET MUSCLES

- Strengthens the abdominals, especially the obliques
- Teaches spinal articulation

ALIGNMENT CUES & OBSTACLES

- Once rolled down, keep the lower back imprinted onto the mat—don't come up into the hip flexion phase of the movement
- Don't let bar twist to and fro—keep it stable
- **Contraindications:** Unstable Sacroiliac joint (can be exacerbated in seated flexion), disc problems in neck, disc dysfunction, osteoporosis

VARIATIONS & PEEL BACKS

- *Roll Downs* are a peel back for this exercise
- Bend knees if you can't get your lower back on the mat

IMAGINE...*you have four points of light making the shape of a rectangle on your abdomen.*

ELLIE SAYS...*"This is a micro-movement... the more micro it is, the more deep in the abs you'll get."*

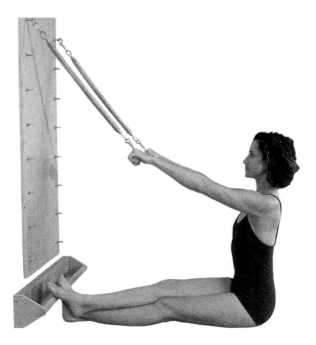

1. Starting Position — *3 repetitions each direction then switch sides*

Hold onto either side of the roll-down bar, thumbs with your fingers, legs straight and hip distance apart, feet touching the wooden dowel. Cross your right leg over your left leg, keeping the right knee soft.

Inhale to prepare; sitting up tall

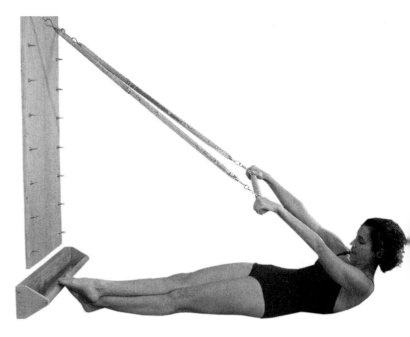

2. Exhale

Roll down the left side of your spine, articulating one vertebra at a time, until your left shoulder is completely flat on the mat, head stays forward and off the mat, squeezing a tangerine. This is your first "point of light."

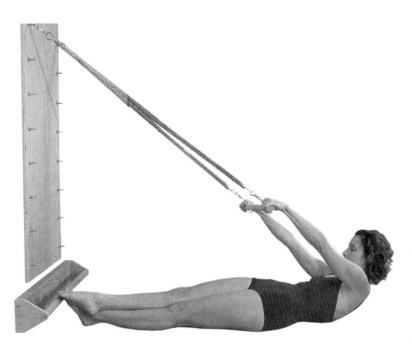

3. Inhale
Roll to your right shoulder. This is your second "point of light."

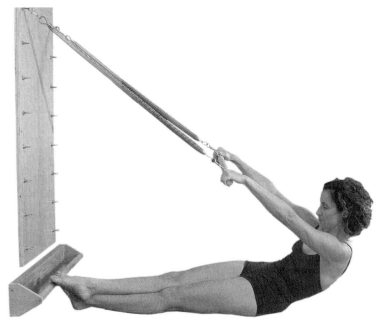

4.
Roll up the right side of your spine slightly; only high enough so that your right low back is still in contact and "imprinted" onto the mat. This is your third "point of light."

5.
Roll to the left side again, imprinting the left low back onto the mat. This is your fourth "point of light."

Continue imprinting these "four points of light" which make a rectangular shape on your torso: Left low back, left shoulder blade, right shoulder blade, right low back. These are small, internal movements.

Repeat 4 cycles and roll up the right side of your spine, stacking up from the base of the spine to return to starting position.

Switch legs and reverse directions.

ROLL-DOWN BAR SET UP

- 6th or 7th eyebolt from the floor
- Adjust 1–2 eyebolts higher if you have a newer Springboard that goes up to 10 or 11

FUNCTIONS & TARGET MUSCLES

- Strengthens the abdominal obliques
- Teaches proper alignment while twisting
- Works hip flexors and spinal extensors

ALIGNMENT CUES & OBSTACLES

- Keep upper trapezius relaxed by engaging low and mid traps
- The rotation of the spine starts with the low ribs and continues up the spine to create a lovely profile of your face—don't just twist neck
- The flow of the movement is: ribs out, ribs in, ribs out
- Focus on isolating the movement to just the rib cage—think "jazz dance warm-up"
- **Contraindications:** Disc dysfunction, osteoporosis

VARIATIONS & PEEL BACKS

- If the leg crossed position causes discomfort in Sacroiliac joint, keep legs uncrossed with feet hip distance apart with knees slightly bent
- **Peel Back:** *Flat Back Roll Down*

IMAGINE...*you are wearing a "beauty pageant banner" across your chest—this will help you feel the diagonal connection of external oblique to opposite internal oblique.*

ELLIE SAYS...*"This one is a little like doing the cabbage patch dance."*

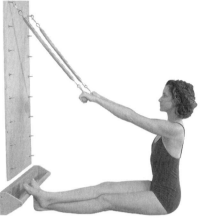

1. Starting Position — *3 repetitions each direction*
Sit facing Springboard, holding onto roll-down bar with hands outside of the springs, thumbs with fingers. Legs are straight with feet hip distance apart, touching the foot bar. Cross right ankle over left ankle, keeping the right knee soft.

Inhale, sitting up tall

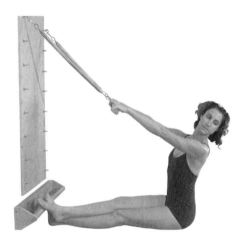

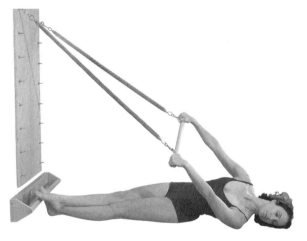

2. Exhale
Rotate rib cage to look over your left shoulder and lift chest slightly, then hinge back at hips, bringing left shoulder down to the mat, grounding your right hip in opposition, making an arcing movement. This is when you imagine your "beauty pageant banner" diagonally crossing your torso from your right hip to your left shoulder.

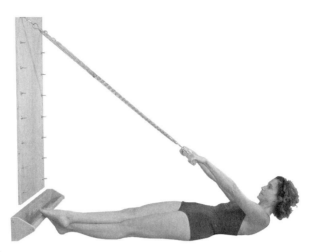

3. Inhale

Keeping head and neck up (squeezing that tangerine, of course) untwist spine bringing your right shoulder onto the mat. Shoulders are square with both scapulae on the mat keeping transversus abdominis engaged (low belly remains hollowed out).

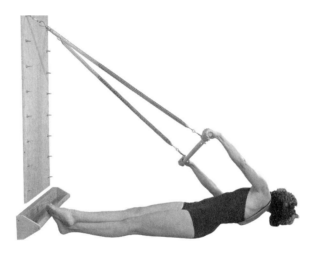

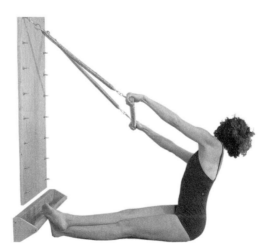

4. Exhale

Twist to right bringing right shoulder off the mat, lift your chest and ribs slightly. Ground left hip and arc back to the start position, feeling the right internal oblique and the left external oblique work as you return to sitting.

Repeat twice more, switch legs, crossing the left leg over the right, and reverse movements.

ROLL-DOWN BAR SET UP

- Roll back bar up to 7–9
- Adjust 1–2 eyebolts higher if you have a newer Springboard that goes up to 10 or 11

FUNCTIONS & TARGET MUSCLES

- Strengthens the abdominals, especially the obliques
- Works upper thoracic spine in deep rotation

ALIGNMENT CUES & OBSTACLES

- You may allow your top hip to drop back a little to allow the shoulders to stay square with the roll-down bar
- Keep the shoulders down away from the ears
- Don't bounce up using momentum—take it slow and use your muscles
- Squeeze the inner thighs together to help stabilize the pelvis
- Press your feet and legs long and away from wall, keeping the legs energized to prevent you from recruiting the quads to help
- **Contraindications:** Disc dysfunction, osteoporosis, neck problems

VARIATIONS & PEEL BACKS

- **Variation:** You can do this exercise with your legs split; top leg forward, bottom leg back. This increases the intensity of the obliques by ensuring proper hip alignment
- **Peel Back:** *Side Body Twist* on Wunda Chair (warms up rotation of upper thoracic spine)

IMAGINE...*the lower half of your body is in a cast and very immobile, then focus, focus, focus on all the work happening at your waist.*

ELLIE SAYS...*"This exercise is a killer for your obliques."*

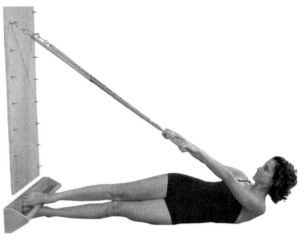

1. Starting Position — *10 repetitions each side*
Hold roll-down bar outside of the springs, thumbs with fingers. Lie on one side with your knees straight, hips long and pelvis stacked and facing the side. The foot bar is between the ankles and toes press away from the wall. Try to keep both arms straight as you twist toward the Springboard, squaring shoulders to the roll back bar.

Inhale to prepare

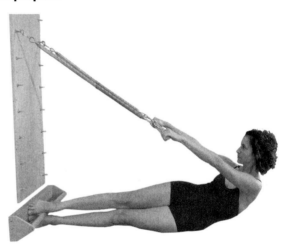

2. Exhale
Pull abdominals toward spine and slowly round halfway up, keeping your hips grounded. Do not jerk your neck to initiate the up movement.

3. Inhale
Roll back, but do not allow head to touch mat between repetitions.

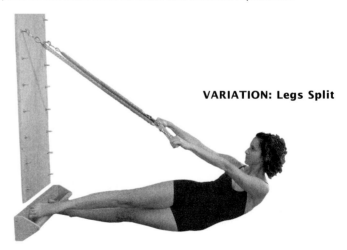

VARIATION: Legs Split

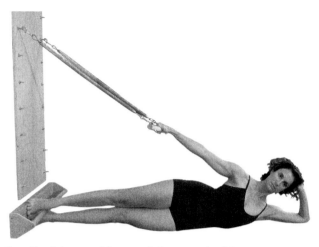

1. Starting Position — *10 repetitions each side*
Lying on side, hold the middle of roll-down bar with top hand, thumb with fingers. Straighten knees with toes pressing into wall, one foot above the foot bar with the other below. Keep both sides of the pelvis stacked with legs slightly in front of you. Use bottom arm to support your head by propping yourself up with your elbow with hand lightly covering the ear.

Inhale to prepare

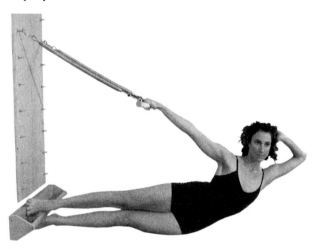

2. Exhale
Pull your abdominals toward your spine and side bend to roll half way up.

3. Inhale
Lower upper torso to the mat, keeping head off the mat between repetitions.

VARIATION: Legs Split

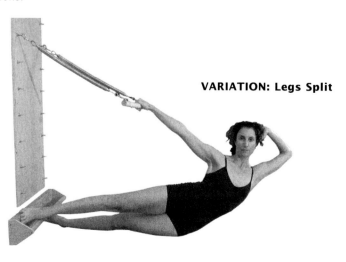

ROLL-DOWN BAR SET UP
- 6th or 7th eyebolt from the floor
- Adjust 1–2 eyebolts higher if you have a newer Springboard that goes up to 10 or 11

FUNCTIONS & TARGET MUSCLES
- Strengthens the abdominal obliques
- Works Quadratus Lumborum
- Great for scoliosis on lengthened side

ALIGNMENT CUES & OBSTACLES
- Make sure your spine stays in slight flexion—don't arch your back (this focuses the work in the abdominals and not the back)
- Keep the shoulders down away from the ears
- Don't bounce up using momentum—take it slow and use your muscles
- Squeeze the inner thighs together to help stabilize the pelvis
- Press your feet and legs long and away from wall, keeping the legs energized to prevent you from recruiting the quads to help
- **Contraindications:** Disc dysfunction on same side (but could help opposite side)

VARIATIONS & PEEL BACKS
- **Variation:** You can do this exercise with your legs split; top leg forward, bottom leg back. This increases the intensity of the obliques by ensuring proper hip alignment.

IMAGINE...*you are closing the space between your ribs and your hips.*

ELLIE SAYS...*"This is also a killer exercise for the obliques. It really tones the waist."*

SUSI SAYS...*"This exercise might seem impossible at first, but you just have to believe in the power of your obliques. It is kind of like clapping to bring Tinker Bell back to life."*

TEASER

ROLL-DOWN BAR SET UP
- 6th or 7th eyebolt from the floor (or higher for more spring assistance)
- Adjust 1–2 eyebolts higher if you have a newer Springboard that goes up to 10 or 11

FUNCTIONS & TARGET MUSCLES
- Strengthens the abdominals and hip flexors
- Works shoulder stabilizers

ALIGNMENT CUES & OBSTACLES
- Allow the bar to stroke the back of the legs as you rise up to the *Teaser*
- **Obstacles:** Tight hamstrings, weak hip flexors
- **Contraindications:** Unstable Sacroiliac joint (can be exacerbated in seated flexion), disc problems in neck, disc dysfunction, osteoporosis, neck problems

VARIATIONS & PEEL BACKS
- **Modification:** To make this exercise easier, do *Teaser* with your legs under the roll-down bar and feet against the wall

IMAGINE...*you are folding in half like a clam closing.*

ELLIE SAYS...*"This is more than just a Teaser, it's a Teaser/Pike."*

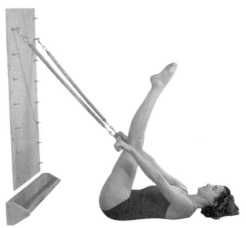

1. Starting Position — *5 repetitions*
Sit facing Springboard and hold roll-down bar with hands outside of the springs, thumbs with fingers. Scoot a few feet away from the Springboard. Lift legs up and bring the roll-down bar behind your legs, making a tight pike position, then lie back on the mat. Knees are straight with feet in Pilates first position.

Inhale to prepare

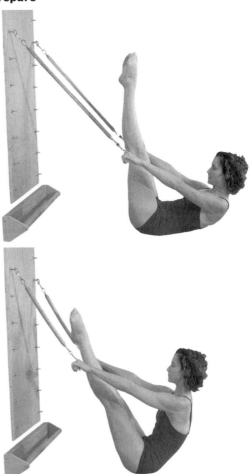

2. Exhale
Lengthen back of neck and left head, squeezing a tangerine under your chin, scooping abdominals towards the spine, and begin to roll up, one vertebra at a time into the Teaser position. Keep shoulders stable as you roll up.

3. Inhale at the top and lift the chest.

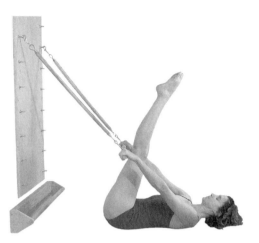

4. Exhale

Roll down, one vertebra at a time, ending with the head relaxed on the mat, returning to starting position.

VARIATION: Teaser/Feet Against Wall

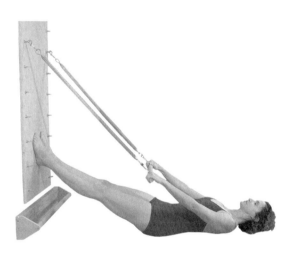

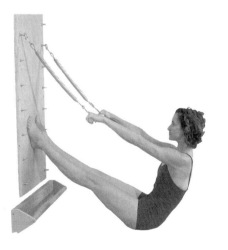

ROLL-DOWN BAR SET UP

- 6th or 7th eyebolt from the floor
- Adjust 1–2 eyebolts higher if you have a newer Springboard that goes up to 10 or 11

FUNCTIONS & TARGET MUSCLES

- Strengthens the abdominals, glutes, triceps and lats
- Stretches the spine and hamstrings

ALIGNMENT CUES & OBSTACLES

- Make sure your spine is very warm before attempting the *Jackknife*, especially in the morning
- **Obstacles:** Tight hamstrings, inflexible spine
- **Contraindications:** Neck injuries, Sacroiliac joint instability, disc dysfunction, osteoporosis

VARIATIONS & PEEL BACKS

- **Modification:** To protect the neck, take out the levitation part and just do a *Rollover*
- **Variations:** Alternate between *Jackknife* and *Teaser* in the pattern—*Jackknife/ Teaser/Jackknife/Teaser*
- **Peel Backs:** *Jackknife* on the mat, *Breathing* on the Cadillac

IMAGINE...you are levitating your hips from the power of your lats pressing down.

ELLIE SAYS..."This is a fun combo with the Teaser."

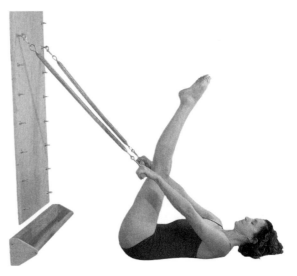

1. Starting Position — *3 repetitions then add the* Teaser *for 3 repetitions*
Sit facing Springboard and hold the roll-down bar with hands outside of the springs, thumbs with fingers. Scoot a few feet away from the Springboard. Lift legs up and bring the roll-down bar behind your legs, making a tight pike position, then lie back on the mat. Legs are straight in Pilates first position.

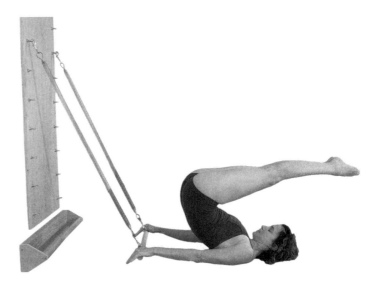

2. Inhale
Lift your hips up and over your head, reaching your toes to the wall behind you. Stop when legs are parallel to the floor and weight is balanced between shoulder blades.

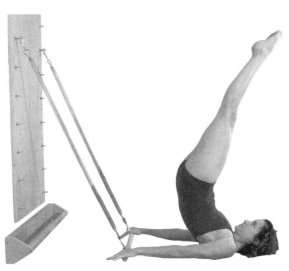

3. Exhale

Using glutes, levitate your hips up toward the sky as you press the roll-down bar down to the floor. Keep weight balanced between shoulder blades.

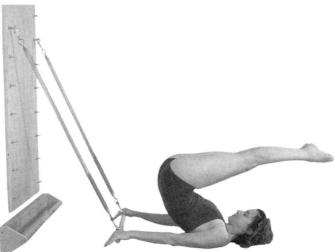

4. Inhale

Fold body in half by lowering legs until they are parallel to the floor, allowing roll-down bar to rise slightly.

Jacknife into Teaser

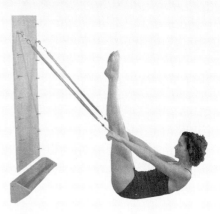

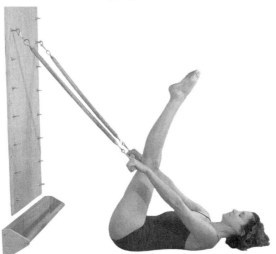

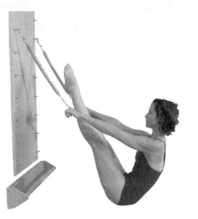

5. Exhale

Roll down one vertebra at a time until pelvis is on the mat and legs are at 90 degrees. Repeat or transition into *Teaser*.

ROLLING LIKE A BALL

ROLL-DOWN BAR SET UP
- 6th or 7th eyebolt from the floor
- Adjust 1–2 eyebolts higher if you have a newer Springboard that goes up to 10 or 11

FUNCTIONS & TARGET MUSCLES
- Strengthens the abdominals, glutes, triceps and lats
- Teaches spinal articulation and coordination

ALIGNMENT CUES & OBSTACLES
- **Obstacle:** Tight spinal extensors
- **Contraindications:** Neck injuries, Sacroiliac joint instability, disc dysfunction, osteoporosis

VARIATIONS & PEEL BACKS
- *Rolling like a Ball* on the mat is a peel back

IMAGINE...*you are a cannon ball.*

ELLIE SAYS...*"This is a real test of your ball-ability."*

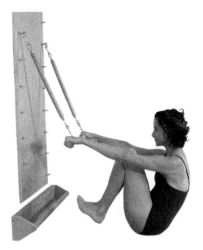

1. Starting Position — *5 repetitions*
Sit facing Springboard and hold roll-down bar with hands outside of the springs, thumbs with fingers. Scoot close to the Springboard, knees bent in toward the chest. Come in to a tight balance point position.

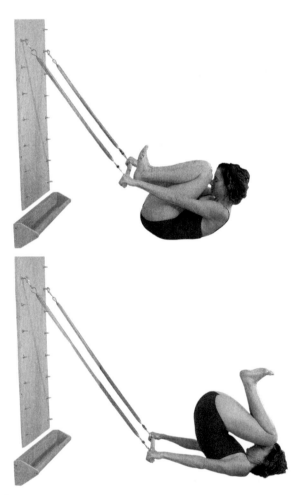

2. Inhale
Maintaining your "small ball" shape, roll back, flexing your feet to fit them through the space under the roll-down bar. Press the roll-down bar down as you lift your hips up, holding the levitation moment, balancing between your shoulder blades.

3. Exhale
Roll forward to the balance point, using abdominal control to prevent your toes from touching the mat, return to starting position.

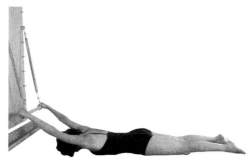

1. Starting Position — *3 sets (9 arm pulls, 9 Swans)*
Lie prone facing the Springboard and place hands on roll-down bar outside of the springs, keeping thumbs with your fingers. You should be an arm's length away from the Springboard. Legs are open more than hip distance apart, with slight external rotation at the hip joint.

Inhale to prepare

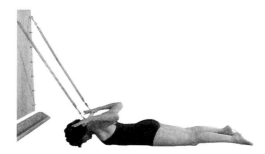

2. Exhale
Keeping the head down and neck relaxed, pull the roll back bar behind your head by bending your elbows to the side. Feel shoulder blades slide down back and to   wards your spine. Think: elbows wide and high.

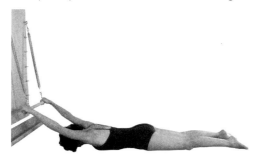

3. Inhale to straighten arms

Repeat arm pull 3 times.

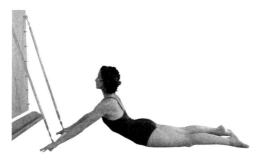

4. Exhale
Pull scapulae down the back as you press the roll-down bar down to the mat, lifting spine off the floor into full extension to come into the Swan position. Keep arms strong and straight, as if you were attempting to stand on them as you rise up. Keep abdominals lifted up off the mat and your pubic bone reaching to the mat as you initiate the Swan. Lift belly and squeeze glutes to protect the low back and SI joint.

5. Inhale
Lower torso to the mat as your arms rise with the springs.

ROLL-DOWN BAR SET UP
- 6th or 7th eyebolt from the floor
- Adjust 1–2 eyebolts higher if you have a newer Springboard that goes up to 10 or 11

FUNCTIONS & TARGET MUSCLES
- Strengthens the lats, triceps, rhomboids, back extensors and glutes
- Opens the chest
- Good for reversing kyphosis and forward head position

ALIGNMENT CUES & OBSTACLES
- Even though the back is going into extension, make sure to keep deep abdominals engaged to support the low back
- As you move into back extension, try to move sequentially through the spine from head to tail
- If you have slim hips, keep inner thighs pulling together
- Having someone hold down the legs allows the glutes to really engage. This is recommended for people with weak abs and glutes and anterior pelvic tilt.
- **Contraindications:** Facet joint problems, stenosis

IMAGINE...*you are pulling yourself out of a pool.*

ELLIE SAYS...*"Another fabulous Swan to try!"*

ROLL-DOWN BAR SET UP

- 6th or 7th eyebolt from the floor
- Adjust 1–2 eyebolts higher if you have a newer Springboard that goes up to 10 or 11

FUNCTIONS & TARGET MUSCLES

- Strengthens lats, triceps, glutes, and hamstrings
- Teaches shoulder stabilization

ALIGNMENT CUES & OBSTACLES

- Make sure the shoulders stay open and don't roll forward
- Make the pulls percussive so that the accent is on the "down" movement
- **Contraindications:** Knee injuries, arthritis of the knees, sensitive knees

VARIATIONS & PEEL BACKS

- **Modification:** If client is uncomfortable kneeling, this can be done standing in Pilates 1st position

IMAGINE...*the pull happens from the back.*

ELLIE SAYS...*"Fun times to be had here."*

MODIFICATION: Standing

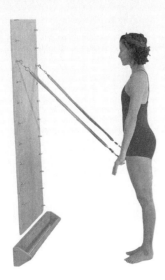

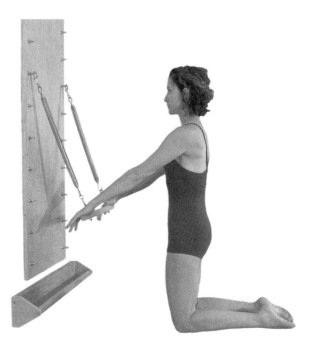

1. Starting Position — *10 repetitions*
Kneel facing the Springboard and hold roll-down bar outside of the springs, keeping thumbs with fingers. You should be an arm's length from the Springboard. Straighten elbows and reach fingers long. You should start with some resistance in the springs. Pitch yourself a wee bit forward, and scoop in belly while tucking pelvis to make the glutes and hamstrings work to stabilize you.

Inhale to prepare

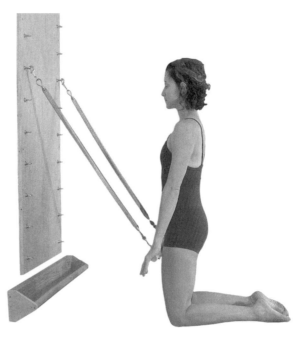

2. Exhale
Keeping elbows straight and shoulders open, pull the roll-down bar toward your thighs. Feel collarbone opening wide.

3. Inhale
Control the bar back up, always keeping some resistance in the bar.

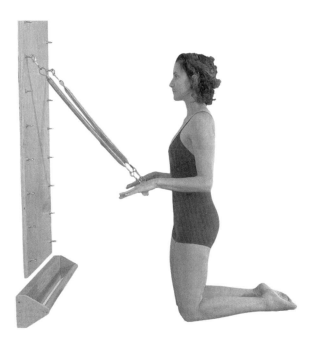

1. Starting Position — *10 repetitions*
Kneel facing the Springboard and hold roll-down bar outside of the springs, keeping thumbs with fingers. Elbows are bent and "glued" to the sides of your body. You should be an arm's length from the Springboard. You should start with some resistance in the springs. Pitch yourself a wee bit forward, while tucking pelvis to make the glutes and hamstrings work to stabilize yourself. Scoop in belly.

Inhale to prepare

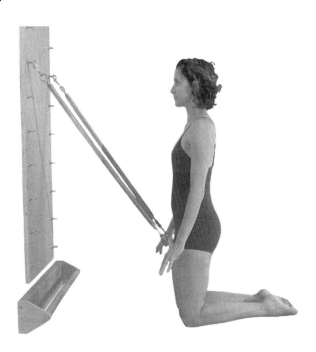

2. Exhale
Keeping the elbows at sides and shoulders open, extend the elbow, pressing the roll-down bar down to your thighs.

3. Inhale
Control the bar back up, always keeping some resistance in the bar.

ROLL-DOWN BAR SET UP
- 6th or 7th eyebolt from the floor
- Adjust 1–2 eyebolts higher if you have a newer Springboard that goes up to 10 or 11

FUNCTIONS & TARGET MUSCLES
- Strengthens triceps, glutes and hamstrings
- Teaches shoulder stabilization

ALIGNMENT CUES & OBSTACLES
- Make sure the shoulders stay open and don't roll forward
- Make the pulls percussive so that the accent is on the "down" movement
- Keep the elbows glued by your sides
- **Contraindications:** Knee injuries, arthritis of the knees, sensitive knees

VARIATIONS & PEEL BACKS
- **Modification:** If you are uncomfortable kneeling, this exercise can be done standing in Pilates 1st position
- **Modification:** If you have narrow shoulders, you can place your hands inside the spring eyebolts on the roll-down bar

IMAGINE...*the movement originates from the stable scapulae.*

ELLIE SAYS...*"This exercise is more about stabilization than tricep work. Motor the exercise from the mid-back."*

MODIFICATION: Standing

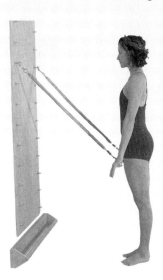

ROLL-DOWN BAR SET UP

- 6th or 7th eyebolt from the floor
- Adjust 1–2 eyebolts higher if you have a newer Springboard that goes up to 10 or 11

FUNCTIONS & TARGET MUSCLES

- Stretches the quads
- Teaches torso stabilization

ALIGNMENT CUES & OBSTACLES

- Be careful of your knees—this is a very loaded stretch!
- **Contraindications:** Knee injuries, arthritis of the knees, sensitive knees

VARIATIONS & PEEL BACKS

- Keep the movement small at first, and know that the further back you hinge, the more stretch you'll feel

IMAGINE..._you are a rigid board as you hinge back._

ELLIE SAYS..._"This exercise can hurt your knees...be aware. If it hurts—stop."_

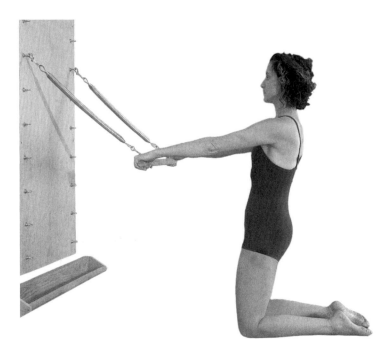

1. Starting Position — *2 times flat back, 2 times arch back*
Kneel facing the Springboard and hold onto the roll-down bar outside of the springs, thumbs with fingers. You should be an arm's length from the Springboard. Reach your arms forward, staying in resistance.

Inhale to prepare

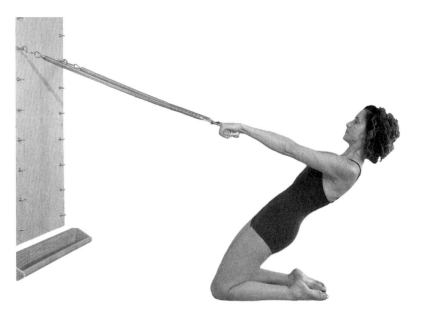

2. Exhale
Keeping the arms straight and shoulders open, hinge back from the knees, keeping your spine stable. Don't allow the ribs to pop open—use your abdominals.

3. Inhale
Rise back up to the upright kneeling position.

Repeat hinge 2 times.

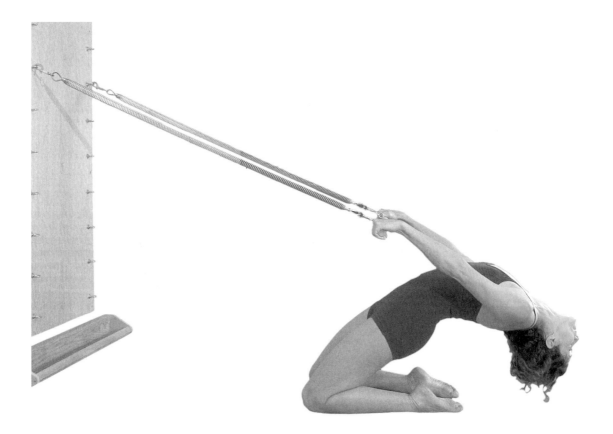

4. Exhale
On the third hinge, go all the back, then arch the back, allowing the head to fully release backward.

5. Inhale
Rise back up, lifting from the chest and sequence the spine back to neutral, flowing up like a rising wave. Do not repeat the arch variation.

ROLL-DOWN BAR SET UP

- 6th or 7th eyebolt from the floor
- Adjust 1–2 eyebolts higher if you have a newer Springboard that goes up to 10 or 11

FUNCTIONS & TARGET MUSCLES

- Stretches the quads
- Teaches spinal articulation and coordination
- Strengthens the glutes, hamstrings, triceps

ALIGNMENT CUES & OBSTACLES

- When returning to the starting position, really use the glutes to keep the pelvis from moving behind the knees while stacking up the spine
- **Contraindications:** Knee injuries, arthritis of the knees, sensitive knees

VARIATIONS & PEEL BACKS

- Keep the hinge back small at first, and increase range of motion as you become more comfortable with the exercise

IMAGINE...*you are a Halloween kitty.*

ELLIE SAYS...*"This is a crazy cat."*

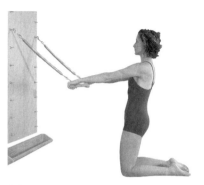

1. Starting Position — *3 repetitions*
Kneel facing the Springboard and hold onto roll-down bar outside of the springs, thumbs with fingers. You should be an arm's length from the Springboard. Extend your arms forward, staying in resistance.

Inhale to prepare

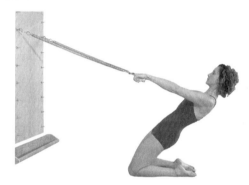

2. Exhale
Keeping the elbows straight and shoulders open, hinge back from the knees, keeping your spine stable; don't allow the ribs to pop—use your upper abdominals.

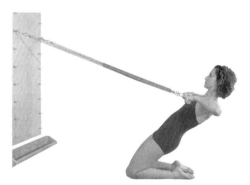

3. Inhale
Pull the bar in toward your chest, bending the elbows wide to the sides.

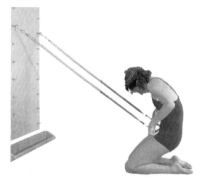

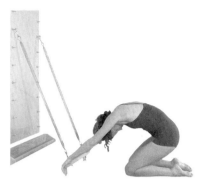

4. Exhale

Stroke your body with the roll back bar, pressing it down your chest, then your thighs, and then toward the floor as you dive underneath a wave with your head, snaking the spine forward in flexion from the head, then follow with the upper back, and then the lower back.

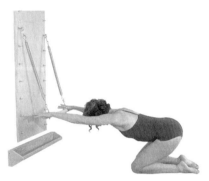

5. Inhale

Come up for air, lifting the head above the wave, allowing the spine to follow into extension, arms long and parallel to the floor, sticking your tail out.

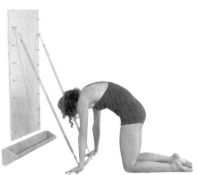

6. Exhale

In one smooth movement, press the roll back bar to the floor as you come into "Halloween kitty," on all fours, entire spine flexed and rounded, pelvis tucked, glutes squeezing, belly scooped.

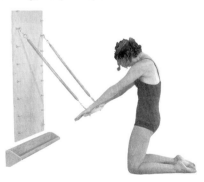

7. Inhale

Controlling the roll-down bar, slowly lift the arms off the mat while stacking up the spine, keeping the hips on top of the knees as you come back to the starting position.

ROLL-DOWN BAR SET UP

- 6th–8th eyebolt from the floor, depending on height of person—the taller the person, the higher the roll-down bar
- Adjust 1–2 eyebolts higher if you have a newer Springboard that goes up to 10 or 11

FUNCTIONS & TARGET MUSCLES

- Strengthens triceps, quads and glutes

ALIGNMENT CUES & OBSTACLES

- Keep your shoulders pulling down the back as you extend your arms
- Keep elbows aligned with hands; don't let them open out

VARIATIONS & PEEL BACKS

- **Modification:** If client has narrow shoulders, try placing hands inside springs on roll-down bar

IMAGINE..._your elbows are fixed by a rod running through the center so you are pivoting around a stable elbow joint._

ELLIE SAYS..._"Work the dingle dangle while you work the legs."_

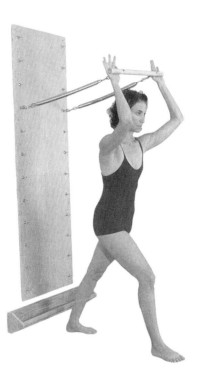

1. Starting Position — *8 to 10 repetitions each side*

Stand facing away the Springboard, hold inside the springs on the roll-down bar, elbows bent and aligned with hands and shoulders. Come into a runner's lunge, bending front knee to a 90 degree angle, the back heel lifted to allow hips to maintain square-ness.

Inhale to prepare

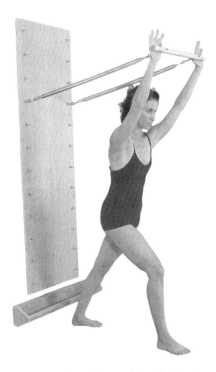

2. Exhale

Extend elbows so arms are straight, reaching the bar forward.

3. Inhale

Control arms back to starting position.

Repeat 8–10 extensions and switch legs.

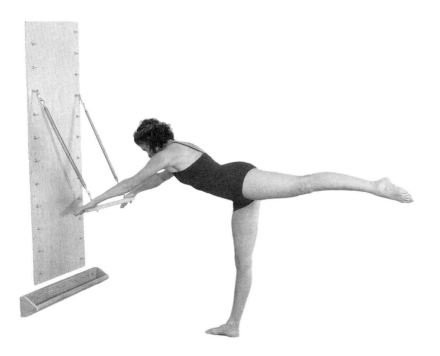

1. Starting Position — *10 repetitions each side*

Stand facing the Springboard, holding the ends of the roll-down bar, thumbs with your fingers. Scoot far enough away from the Springboard so that you will still be in resistance when you extend your arms forward. Stand on one leg and lift the other leg back behind you as you lean forward, arms straight, pressing down slightly into spring resistance. The standing leg is parallel, while the extended leg is in turn out. Keep hips square.

Inhale to prepare

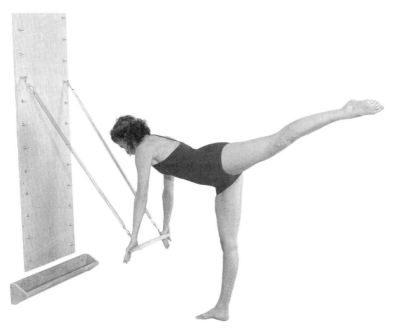

2. Exhale

Press the roll-down bar down toward your standing thigh, just like a *Lat Pull*, while you lift the extended leg up in the air. Every time you pull the roll-down bar down, the back leg lifts up slightly.

ROLL-DOWN BAR SET UP
- 8th or 9th eyebolt from the floor
- Adjust 1–2 eyebolts higher if you have a newer Springboard that goes up to 10 or 11

FUNCTIONS & TARGET MUSCLES
- Strengthens lats, triceps, hamstrings and glutes
- Teaches balance and control

ALIGNMENT CUES & OBSTACLES
- Keep your shoulders pulling down the back as you do your lat pull

VARIATIONS & PEEL BACKS
- **Peel Back:** *Standing Lat Pull*
- **Variation:** Try "Warrior 3" with legs in parallel, hip points facing down to the floor

IMAGINE...as you pull the bar, your leg automatically pulses up.

ELLIE SAYS..."This is like the Arabesque on the Reformer, but harder!"

PILATES SQUAT

ROLL-DOWN BAR SET UP

- 7th–9th eyebolt from the floor, depending on height of person
- Adjust 1–2 eyebolts higher if you have a newer Springboard that goes up to 10 or 11

FUNCTIONS & TARGET MUSCLES

- Strengthens quads, hamstrings, glutes and biceps

ALIGNMENT CUES & OBSTACLES

- Keep your knees aiming over your 3rd toes
- Keep the shoulders open and shoulder blades pulling down the back

VARIATIONS & PEEL BACKS

- **See opposite page**

IMAGINE...*you are sitting down on an invisible chair.*

IMAGINE...*your arm starts at your shoulder blade.*

ELLIE SAYS...*"Great for the bootay."*

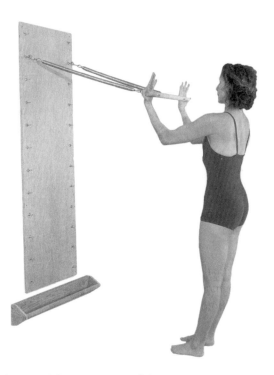

1. Starting Position — *8 repetitions*
Stand facing the Springboard, with legs hip distance apart, holding the ends of the roll-down bar with palms facing you, and bend your elbows to a 90 degree angle, keeping the upper arm at the height of the shoulder. Your arms should be pulling into the resistance.

Inhale to prepare

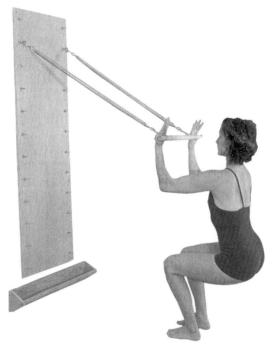

2. Exhale
Maintaining the 90 degree angle at the elbow, press into your heels and bend your knees, coming down into a squat, no lower than 90 degree angle at your knees. Stick your butt out a little.

Hold for one full breath and then come back up.

VARIATION: Squat with Arm Pulls

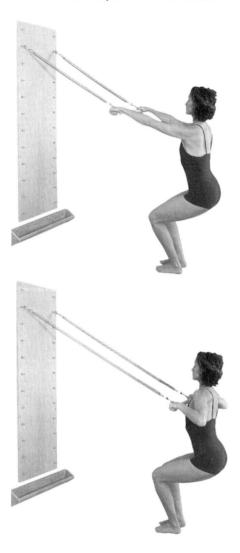

VARIATIONS & PEEL BACKS

- **Variation:** *Squat with Arm Pulls*
  Try either squat holding the bar with hands on top and do 8 arm pulls, pulling elbows wide to the sides while holding your squat.

- **Variation:** *QL Stretch*
  Holding outside of roll-down bar, walk back so that there is some tension on the springs and turn 90 degrees so that your feet and hips are square to the side wall, while your shoulders are square to the Springboard. Bend knees and flex lower spine until you feel a stretch in the side of your lower back.

- **Variation:** (not shown) Squat with knees and feet together (Utkatasana in yoga). Try the squat holding the bar with hands on top, and keeping knees and feet squeezing together, bend knees to a 90 degree angle and lean slightly forward from torso. Allow pelvis to be neutral or even slightly anterior (stick your butt out a little) and then pull up from the pelvic floor and low belly to lengthen low back. Hold for 10–30 seconds or add arm pulls above.

- **Variation:** *2nd Position* (not shown)
  Legs turned out and wide apart.

VARIATION: QL Stretch

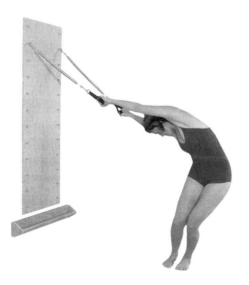

JUMPING

ROLL-DOWN BAR SET UP

- The highest eyebolt you can reach

FUNCTIONS & TARGET MUSCLES

- Strengthens quads, hamstrings, glutes, biceps
- Conditions the lower limbs for explosive movements
- Aerobic conditioning

ALIGNMENT CUES & OBSTACLES

- Keep your knees aiming over each of your 3rd toes
- Keep the shoulders open and shoulder blades pulling down the back
- Stick your butt out slightly when you land to maximize the use of the gluteus maximus

VARIATIONS & PEEL BACKS

- **Variation:** Jumping in second position—legs open wide and turned out

IMAGINE..._you are jumping back into the abyss._

ELLIE SAYS..._"This one will really get your butt strong."_

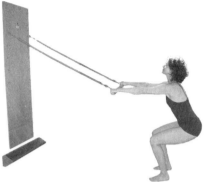

1. Starting Position — *10 jumps per set, 3 sets*
Stand facing the Springboard, with legs hip distance apart and feet in parallel, holding the roll-down bar with palms down, arms straight. Bend your knees into a squat, leaning your torso forward slightly and allowing your butt to stick out a little. Start with a squat prep.

Inhale to prepare

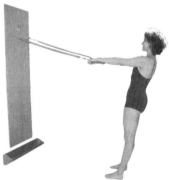

2. Exhale
Extend legs and hips, pushing forward from glutes and hamstrings, leaning back slightly. Repeat 5–10 times.

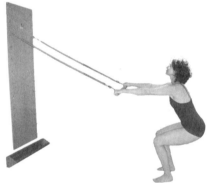

3. Inhale
Start from squat.

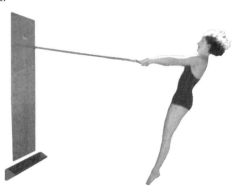

4. Exhale
Jump up and back on the diagonal, into the resistance, and then land back in the squat.

Repeat 10 times. Rest and repeat cycle again 2 more times.

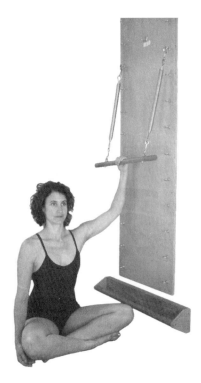

ROLL-DOWN BAR SET UP
- 8th or 9th eyebolt from the floor
- Adjust 1–2 eyebolts higher if you have a newer Springboard that goes up to 10 or 11

FUNCTIONS & TARGET MUSCLES
- Strengthens lats
- Trains proper shoulder abduction

ALIGNMENT CUES & OBSTACLES
- Keep elbow in line with ear
- Pull scapula down the back to initiate the movement of the arm

VARIATIONS & PEEL BACKS
- **Peel Back:** *One Arm Lat Pull* on Cadillac

ELLIE SAYS... *"Use the lat, not the bicep"*

1. Starting Position — *5 repetitions*
Sit cross-legged in profile to the Springboard, and hold the middle of the bar with palm facing you, elbow aligned with ear. Sit up tall.

Inhale to prepare

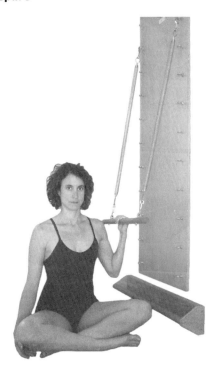

2. Exhale
Pull the scapula down the back, then pull the bar down as far as possible, keeping elbow in line with hand.

3. Inhale and hold

4. Exhale
Pull scapula down the back as you return to starting position.

SEATED CHICKEN WINGS

ROLL-DOWN BAR SET UP
- Springs on the highest eyebolt for all Springboards

FUNCTIONS & TARGET MUSCLES
- Strengthens lats
- Stretches pectorals and chest
- Trains proper shoulder abduction

ALIGNMENT CUES & OBSTACLES
- Sit up tall
- Keep elbows in a two dimensional plane with hands behind your head
- Initiate movement of the arms in both directions by pulling the scapulae down the back

VARIATIONS & PEEL BACKS
- **Peel Back:** *Chicken Wings* on roller or Reformer

IMAGINE... *you are doing a lat pull at the gym—but with more grace.*

ELLIE SAYS... *"Yummy stretch for the chest!"*

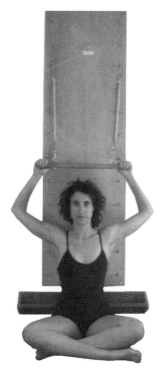

1. Starting Position — *8 to 10 repetitions*
Sit cross-legged with the back close to the Springboard and hold onto the ends of the roll-down bar, palms facing forward. Sit up tall.

Inhale to prepare

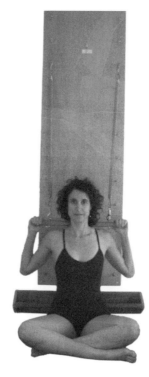

2. Exhale
Pull the scapulae down the back, then pull the bar down behind your head keeping elbows wide and open.

3. Inhale and hold

4. Exhale
Pull scapulae down the back as you return to the starting position.

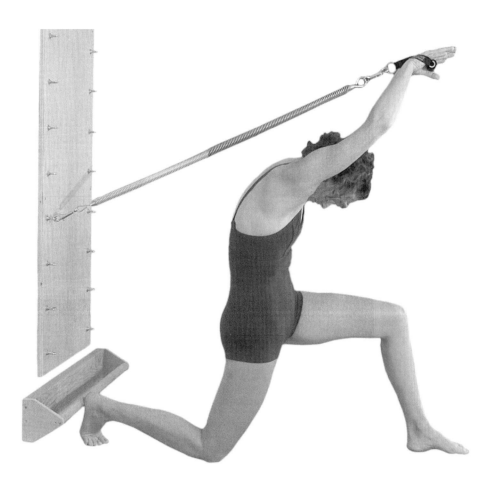

Arm Springs are an excellent way to strengthen and stabilize the shoulder girdle, build muscle tone in the upper body, and teach coordination.

The arm springs pictured in this book are short yellow springs with neoprene handles attached. They are the same springs that are used with the Roll–Down Bar. These springs are quite heavy and not appropriate for many people, especially smaller women and people with unstable shoulders. You can use long yellow springs, often referred to as leg springs, and that will give a greater sense of ease than the short yellow springs. In the last couple of years, I have started replacing all my arms springs with 31" stroops. They come in blue (medium weight) or yellow (light weight). Stoops are black, cloth covered bungees, which are a great substitute for arm springs.

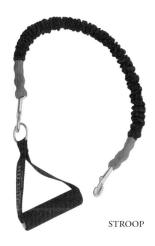

STROOP

Some of the Springboard Arm Springs exercises are identical to Reformer exercises; i.e. Seated Rowing Series, Kneeling Series, *Hundred, Coordination,* etc. Others are classical Cadillac exercises; i.e. Standing Arm Series.

ARM SPRINGS SET UP

- 2nd or 3rd eyebolt from the floor
- Adjust 1–2 eyebolts higher if you have a newer Springboard that goes up to 10 or 11

FUNCTIONS & TARGET MUSCLES

- Strengthens lats while stabilizing pelvis and rib cage
- Peel back for *Overhead*
- Teaches *Doorframe Arms*

ALIGNMENT CUES & OBSTACLES

- To avoid overworking pec major, do not allow shoulder to internally rotate so far that glenohumeral joint loses contact with mat
- Feel scapula sliding down back as arms move
- Keep elbows and wrists straight
- If pecs are overworking, have client widen arms and bend elbows slightly
- If client has flat kyphotic curve, cue them to feel spine between the scapula making contact with mat

VARIATIONS & PEEL BACKS

- **Variation:** *Angel Wings:* (Beginning) (not shown) Start with arms out to sides and parallel to floor, palms toward ceiling. Pull arms to sides on exhale and control back to start position on inhale (like making angels in the snow)
- As client gets stronger, increase spring setting
- Use tabletop leg position to increase abdominal work (but do not allow lumbar spine to hyperextend)
- As a peel back for *The Hundreds,* add upper abdominal curl as arms pull down

IMAGINE... *your neck is growing away from your body as arms pull down.*

ELLIE SAYS... *"Scapulae are the feet of your arms and you're standing on your scapulae."*

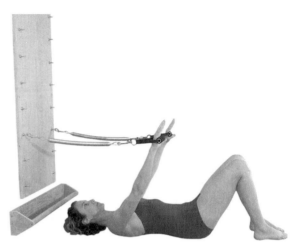

1. Starting Position — *5 repetitions*
Lie on your back with your head close to the Springboard. Hands in handles with fingers reaching toward the sky. Back is wide with entire scapula making contact with the mat. Starting position should be in slight spring resistance.

Inhale to prepare

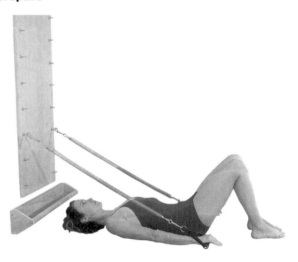

2. Exhale
Engage abdominals while pulling arms down toward carriage until palms make contact with mat.

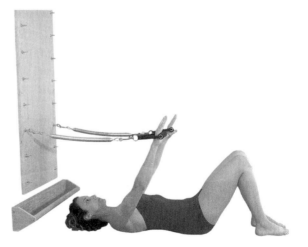

3. Inhale
Arms rise back to starting position (not home).

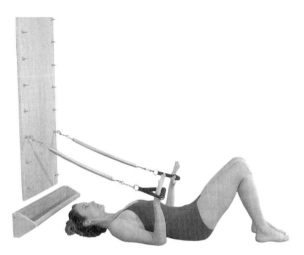

1. Starting Position — *5 repetitions*
Lie on your back with your head close to the Springboard. Start with elbows glued to your side, elbows bent to 90 degrees, palms forward with long fingers.

Inhale to prepare

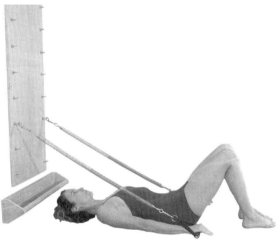

2. Exhale
Extend arms to floor.

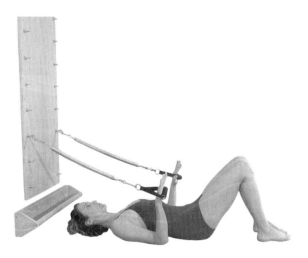

3. Inhale
Control back to start position on inhale, keeping shoulders rotated open, scapulae pressing onto mat.

ARM SPRINGS SET UP
- 2nd or 3rd eyebolt from the floor
- Adjust 1–2 eyebolts higher if you have a newer Springboard that goes up to 10 or 11

FUNCTIONS & TARGET MUSCLES
- Strengthens triceps while stabilizing pelvis and rib cage

ALIGNMENT CUES & OBSTACLES
- Feel scapula sliding down back as arms move
- Keep wrists and fingers long
- If client has flat kyphotic curve, cue them to feel spine between the scapula making contact with mat

VARIATIONS & PEEL BACKS
- As client gets stronger, increase spring setting
- Use tabletop leg position to increase abdominal work (but do not allow lumbar spine to hyperextend)

ARM SPRINGS SET UP

- 2nd or 3rd eyebolt from the floor
- Adjust 1–2 eyebolts higher if you have a newer Springboard that goes up to 10 or 11

FUNCTIONS & TARGET MUSCLES

- To warm up the body
- Strengthens abdominal muscles, hip flexors, deep neck flexors, and lats
- Challenges coordination—pumping arms in rhythm with breath while maintaining torso stability
- Teaches percussive breathing

ALIGNMENT CUES & OBSTACLES

- On each round of exhales, deepen abdominal engagement and come up higher to maintain Pilates abdominal position
- Do not just use rectus abdominis—keep pulling navel to spine to protect the low back
- Maintain doorframe arms while pumping
- Keep upper body stable—do not let upper body rock with arm pumps
- To keep neck relaxed, look to right for one set of breaths and then to left for the next, but do not allow scapulae to touch mat or torso to rock with head
- **Obstacles:** Weak abs and weak hip flexors
- **Contraindications:** Neck injuries, osteoporosis

VARIATIONS & PEEL BACKS

- Lumbar spine is deeply imprinted on mat and low glutes are engaged
- **Variation:** (not shown) Can perform *Frog Extensions* with legs straightening on each set of exhales to relax hip flexors

IMAGINE..._you are cradling a bowling ball with your spine—so if you're over using your rectus you're going to pop the ball off your torso._

IMAGINE..._your sternum is anchored to the mat and you're "hatch-backing" the upper back around this anchor._

ELLIE SAYS..._"Traditionally The Hundreds is a 'warm up' exercise because it gets the blood circulating."_

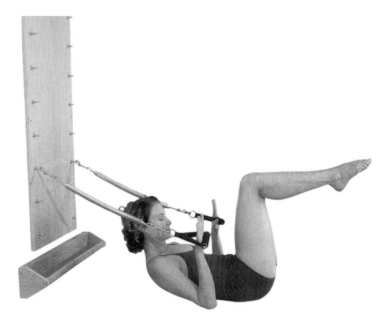

1. Starting position — *10 sets of 10 breaths*
Lie on your back with your head close to the Springboard. Place hands in handles bringing elbows to the sides of your body with elbows bent to 90 degrees. Legs are in tabletop position.

Inhale to prepare

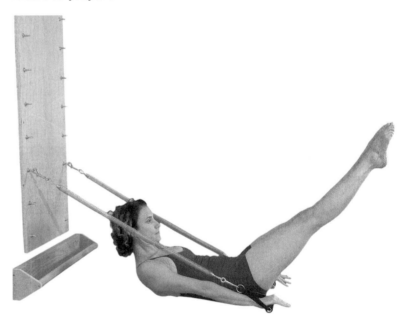

Exhale
Roll up to *Pilates abdominal position* while pressing arms to the mat (*Tricep Press*).

2. Inhale through nose, either smoothly or percussively, for 5 arm pumps—pumping the entire arm.

3. Exhale percussively for 5 arm pumps.

Complete 10 sets of 10 pumps to make 100.

Beginning Variation

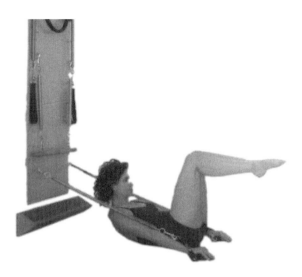

VARIATIONS & PEEL BACKS

- **Beginning:** Use tabletop leg position and maintain neutral spine
- **Intermediate:** Knees straight, legs slightly lower than 90 degrees, hips in slight external rotation making feet in the Pilates "V" (this favors the psoas for hip flexion), lumbar spine is scooped slightly past neutral
- **Advanced:** Knees straight and legs low as possible maintaining abdominal scoop

Intermediate Variation

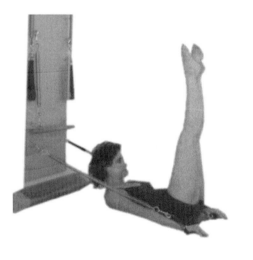

ARM SPRINGS SET UP

- 2nd or 3rd eyebolt from the floor
- Adjust 1–2 eyebolts higher if you have a newer Springboard that goes up to 10 or 11

FUNCTIONS & TARGET MUSCLES

- Strengthens abdominal muscles, hips flexors, deep neck flexors, and triceps
- Challenges client coordination—legs moving independently of arms

ALIGNMENT CUES & OBSTACLES

- Perform this exercise with finesse and control with accent on IN motion as legs open and close
- Maintain *Pilates abdominal positioning*—no decrease in spinal flexion, no dropping or juicing the imaginary fruit between chin and chest
- **Contraindications:** Neck injuries, osteoporosis

VARIATIONS & PEEL BACKS

- It is easier on the neck to keep it flexed rather than lifting and lowering the head with each repetition—if client has neck issues have them try the exercise keeping head down and just moving arms and legs, then add 1 or 2 repetitions with head raising into *Pilates abdominal position*
- To challenge the abdominals: when knees are straight add *Running* or *Scissor* legs from *Leg Spring* series—legs go only as low as abdominal scoop can be maintained and lumbar spine stays slightly flexed
- **Peel Backs:** Tricep pulls, then add tricep pulls with upper abdominal curl

IMAGINE...*you are very coordinated.*

ELLIE SAYS...*"Cue it like this: Extend ... Open ... Close ... Knees ... Arms."*

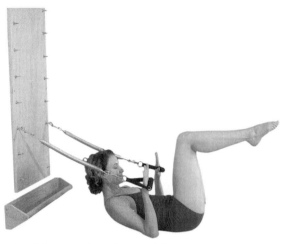

1. Starting Position — *5 or 6 repetitions*
Lie on your back with your head close to the Springboard, hands in handles with elbow bent to 90 degrees and fingertips toward ceiling, upper arms glued to sides, legs in tabletop position.

Inhale to prepare

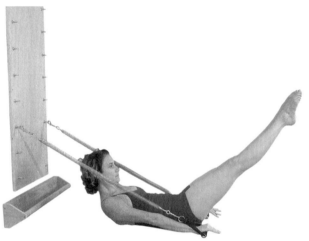

2. Percussive Exhale
Extend arms and legs into *"Hundred"* position keeping belly scooped in and lower back flat on the mat.

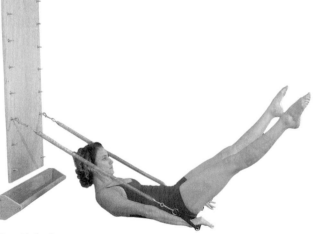

3. Percussive Exhale
Open legs slightly wider than hips.

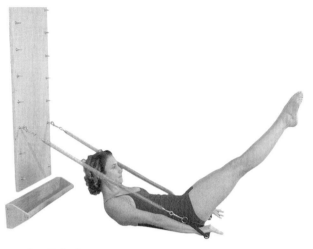

4. Percussive Exhale
Close legs.

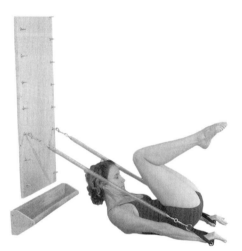

5. Percussive Exhale
Bend knees toward chest and do small hip-up.

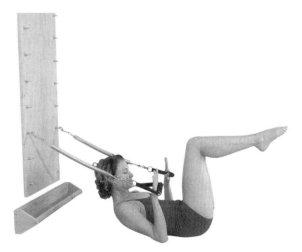

6. Inhale
Bend elbows to 90 degrees—elbows stay on mat—maintaining *Pilates Abdominal Position.*

HUG A TREE

ARM SPRINGS SET UP

- 2nd or 3rd eyebolt from the floor
- Adjust 1–2 eyebolts higher if you have a newer Springboard that goes up to 10 or 11

FUNCTIONS & TARGET MUSCLES

- Strengthens deltoids and pectoralis major
- Works abdominals and postural muscles
- Teaches scapular stabilization with humeral motion (mid trapezius, serratus anterior, rhomboids)

ALIGNMENT CUES & OBSTACLES

- Keep head aligned over pelvis in excellent sitting posture while moving arms
- Sit right on sits bones—no slouching behind them or arching in front of them
- Feel chest and back staying wide and stable as arms move
- Reach through pinky finger to encourage the serratus anterior to work
- If client is unable to sit up straight in crossed legged position place them on a moon box, mat, or pillow
- As arms return to starting position do not let elbows move behind torso—this will pinch shoulder blades and force pecs to initiate the next "hug"
- Think "ballet arms"

VARIATIONS & PEEL BACKS

- To increase difficulty, sit with legs straight in front of you
- To work arm strength, use red spring

IMAGINE...*you're Shiva and you have 2 extra sets of arms, with one set attached to your scapulae and the other set attached to your rib cage. Hug the tree with all 6 of your arms and the tree will feel the love.*

ELLIE SAYS...*"Romana used to call this Hug Pavarotti."*

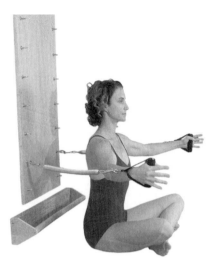

1. Starting Position — *6 repetitions*

Sit cross-legged facing away from the Springboard with back close to it. Hands in handles with arms to sides, hands and elbows slightly lower than shoulders. Elbows are slightly rounded. Arms are slightly in front of torso. You should be able to see your elbows with your peripheral vision. These are "ballet arms."

Inhale and lengthen spine

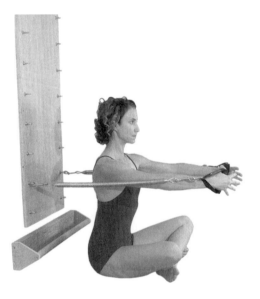

2. Inhale

Open arms to starting position, growing ever taller in spine.

After 3 repetitions reverse the breathing so the arms pull together on inhale for 3 more repetitions. Breathe wide into the lateral ribs as you initiate the hug.

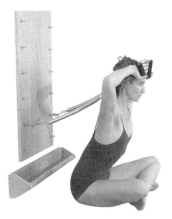

1. Starting Position — *6 repetitions (3 of each variation)*
Sit cross-legged with hands in handles, facing away but close to the Springboard. Salute forehead with elbows bent, and index fingers, touching eyebrows with palms facing out. Torso is pitched forward about 20 degrees from upright.

Inhale to prepare

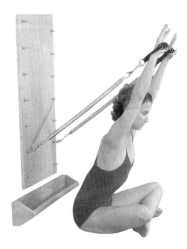

2. Exhale
Straighten elbows while stabilizing the scapulae so they don't elevate. Arms straighten to doorframe position on the line of the body. Hands are even with or wider than shoulders.

3. Inhale
Elbows bend and fingers return to eyebrows. Repeat 3 times.

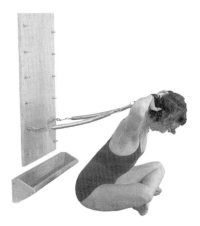

4. Exhale
Drop head forward bringing hands behind head and salute the Pilates Goddess from this position (like you're shaving off the back of your head).

5. Inhale
Return to starting position with control.

ARM SPRINGS SET UP
- 2nd or 3rd eyebolt from the floor
- Adjust 1–2 eyebolts higher if you have a newer Springboard that goes up to 10 or 11

FUNCTIONS & TARGET MUSCLES
- Strengthens triceps and deltoids
- Teaches shoulder girdle stability

ALIGNMENT CUES & OBSTACLES
- Keep shoulders wide and scapulae sliding down back—DO NOT OVERUSE UPPER TRAPS
- If it is difficult to keep shoulders down, allow arms to widen as they extend—saluting more toward the side than the front (work to narrow the salute)
- Be careful to keep the head and neck in line with the spine (no forward head)
- **Obstacles:** Tight upper traps, tight lats (inhibit shoulder flexion and create sensation of compression in shoulder girdle and neck), tight hips and/or tight low back (make it difficult to hinge forward—in this case have client sit on mat, pillow, or moon box)
- **Contraindication:** Clients with carpal tunnel and upper quarter Repetitive Stress Injury issues because it is very difficult to not overuse upper traps and levator scapula

VARIATIONS & PEEL BACKS
- To make this exercise more difficult, once client is able to keep shoulder girdle stable, drop head forward bringing hands behind head and salute from this position—3 repetitions of each variation
- **Peel Backs:** *Double Lat Pulls* on the Cadillac (both versions)

IMAGINE...*you are saluting the Pilates Goddess.*

SUSI SAYS...*"I rarely see this exercise done correctly. So don't teach it to your clients until they can stabilize their shoulders while raising their arms above their heads seated upright. That pitch forward truly increases the difficulty of this exercise."*

MODIFIED FRONT ROWING

ARM SPRINGS SET UP

- 2nd or 3rd eyebolt from the floor
- Adjust 1–2 eyebolts higher if you have a newer Springboard that goes up to 10 or 11

FUNCTIONS & TARGET MUSCLES

- Strengthens deltoids
- Strengthens abdominals and postural muscles
- Teaches scapular stabilization and works mid traps, serratus anterior, rhomboids

ALIGNMENT CUES & OBSTACLES

- With every inhale, lengthen spine and maintain that length with every exhale—using abdominals, of course
- Feel scapulae sliding down back as arms raise
- Feel pinkies cut through space as you lower arms to sides
- Feel lats stretch as arms rise above head
- Keep hands in peripheral vision as arms lower to sides
- Do not sacrifice rib cage stability to align arms with spine—"don't let ribs poke out"
- **Obstacles:** Tight lats and upper traps

VARIATIONS & PEEL BACKS

- If client is unable to sit up straight in crossed-legged position, place them on a moon box, mat, or pillow
- Widen arms if necessary to keep shoulders down while raising arms above head
- Peel back for *Front Rowing Combo*

IMAGINE...*your head is poking through the clouds every time you lower your arms.*

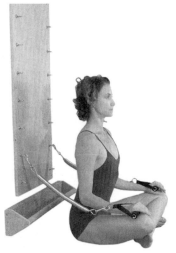

1. Starting Position — *4 repetitions*
Sit cross-legged facing away from Springboard with back close to it. Hands in handles resting on knees.

Inhale, lengthen spine.

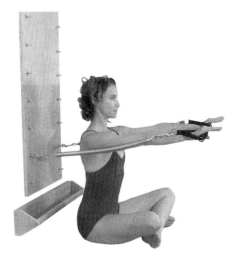

2. Exhale
Pull abdominals toward spine, stabilize scapulae and straighten arms while raising them to 90 degrees—shoulder height ("shave off the tops of the knees").

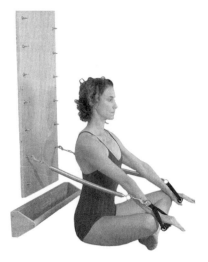

3. Inhale
Lengthen spine while lowering arms, bringing hands back to knees. Keep arms straight.

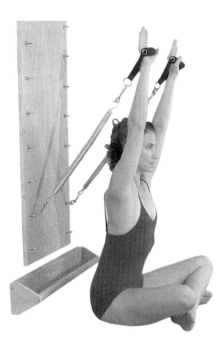

4. Exhale
Pull abdominals toward spine, stabilize scapulae and straighten elbows while raising arms above head (widen arms if necessary to keep shoulders away from ears)—making one long line from tailbone to top of head.

5. Inhale
Just lengthen the spine and widen the back, feeling the last stretch.

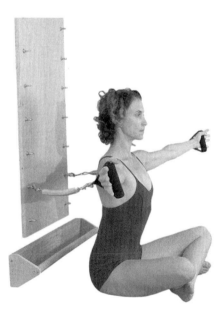

6. Exhale
Spine grows taller as arms open to sides, as if you are cutting through the air with your pinky fingers.

7. Inhale
"Sneak" hands back to top of knees to return to starting position.

ARM SPRINGS SET UP

- 2nd or 3rd eyebolt from the floor
- Adjust 1–2 eyebolts higher if you have a newer Springboard that goes up to 10 or 11

FUNCTIONS & TARGET MUSCLES

- Strengthens shoulder stabilizers
- Stretches lats, spinal erectors and hamstrings
- Challenges coordination and memory

ALIGNMENT CUES & OBSTACLES

- As always keep upper traps as relaxed as possible and keep scapulae stable on a wide back, not elevated toward ears
- Feel energy shooting out of heels when feet are flexed and out of toes when feet are pointed
- Do not collapse to bend forward—lengthen spine as if you were curving over a beach ball
- Do not pop ribs or hyperextend lumbar spine when pitching forward—use those abdominals to keep the spine stable
- **Obstacles:** Tight hamstrings, tight lats, weak psoas
- **Contraindications:** Disc dysfunction, osteoporosis

VARIATIONS & PEEL BACKS

- **Modification:** If client is has very tight hamstrings, teach this exercise with a pillow or mat under their pelvis or with them seated cross-legged
- **Peel Backs:** *Modified Front Rowing, Salute*

IMAGINE...*you are Martha Graham doing her famous C-Curve.*

ELLIE SAYS..."*Since the Advanced Rowing Combos contain intricate movements and complex choreography, they are some of the hardest Pilates exercises to memorize. So practice them regularly until they are emblazoned on your memory.*"

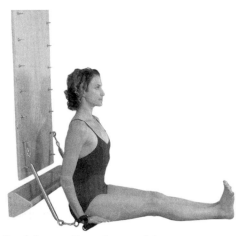

1. Starting Position — *3 or 4 repetitions*
Sit upright with back close to Springboard. Legs are lengthened in front of body with ankles, knees, and inner thighs touching. Place hands in handles with arms by sides and palms resting on mat.

Inhale lengthen spine to prepare

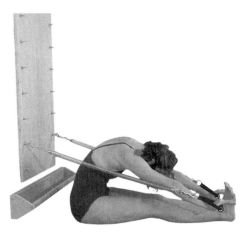

2. Exhale
Flex feet, pull abdominals to spine and bend forward, rounding spine, bringing nose toward knees. Slide hands along carriage reaching arms toward toes.

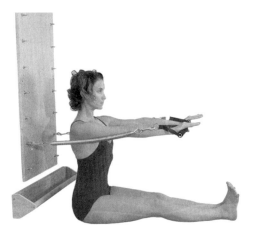

3. Inhale
Stack spine sequentially from tail to head bringing arms up with torso, fingers reach forward with straight elbows. Hands are in line with shoulders and palms remain toward floor. Keep back wide and pecs relaxed. "Ka-chunk" the humerus into the back.

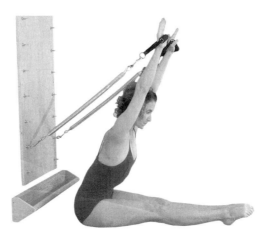

4. Exhale

Point feet and pitch forward, hinging at hips, reaching from base of spine while raising arms up as torso stretches diagonally forward, creating one line from tailbone to fingertips. Torso moves forward and arms reach up, creating the *Salute* position. Keep scapulae stable.

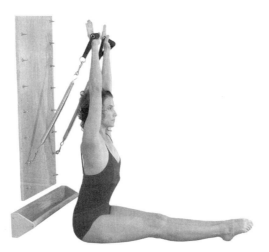

5. Inhale

Bring upper body upright in one piece. Fingers reach toward ceiling with energy shooting out of top of head while shoulders remain connected to back.

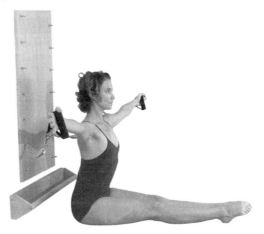

6. Exhale

Leading with pinkies, open arms wide to the sides keeping hands in your peripheral vision. Spine grows taller as arms return to sides with hands resting on the mat.

BACK ROWING ROUND BACK

ARM SPRINGS SET UP

- 2nd or 3rd eyebolt from the floor
- Adjust 1–2 eyebolts higher if you have a newer Springboard that goes up to 10 or 11

FUNCTIONS & TARGET MUSCLES

- Strengthens shoulder stabilizers
- Stretches spinal erectors and works abdominals
- Stretches shoulders and arms
- Challenges coordination and memory

ALIGNMENT CUES & OBSTACLES

- Really use abdominals to resist movement of spine bending forward or rolling up to enhance spine stretch
- In the starting arm position elbows are bent just enough to feel upper back widen without over-engaging pecs weak psoas
- **Contraindications:** Disc dysfunction, osteoporosis

IMAGINE... *you are a bird of prey about to pounce as you complete the final movement of the exercise.*

SUSI SAYS... *"This version of rowing always reminds of the dying swan from the Swan Lake. So perform Round Back Rowing with finesse and a sense of drama."*

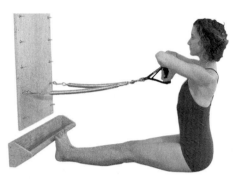

1. Starting Position — *3 repetitions*
Sit upright facing Springboard, legs lengthened and straight in front you. Hold the handles with long arms, then bend the elbows into a diamond shape with top fists coming together. Feet are flexed squeezing together inner thighs.

Inhale and engage low glutes lengthening torso away from pelvis

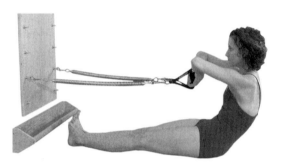

2. Exhale
Pull abdominals to spine, reach through heels, and round lumbar spine, pulling torso behind sits bones, rolling about 1/2 way down. Make sure to maintain the diamond shape as you roll back, pulling on the spring resistance.

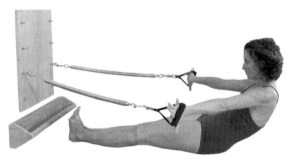

3. Inhale
Maintain C–Curve of spine and open arms to sides by hinging from elbows. Keep scapulae engaged down back.

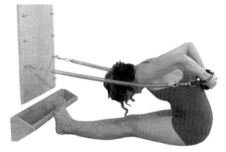

4. Exhale
Increase abdominal engagement, hollowing out the front of the body to bring upper body through arms as they circle around behind the back in a kind of grandiose breaststroke action—the body then begins to fold in half. Reaching arms behind torso, slowly round spine forward, bringing the nose toward the knees and clasping hands behind back, interlacing fingers. Then bend elbows, bringing hands toward body.

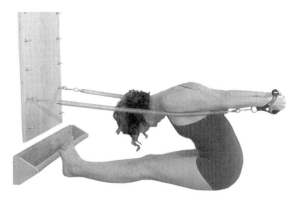

5. Inhale
Straighten arms, rotating the shoulders open, keeping everything else perfectly still. Pull scapulae together.

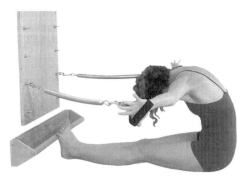

6. Exhale
Release hands without "popping." Circle arms forward, pulling abdominals deeply to spine to round up. Arms continue circling until they are parallel and the back of hands face one another. This is your "bird of prey" moment—really accentuate the thoracic C–Curve.

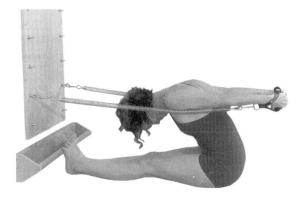

7. Inhale
Stack up from base of spine coming into seated upright position, bending elbows, bringing back of hands together, moving hands toward sternum to create a diamond shape. Squeeze low glutes in preparation to repeat exercise.

BACK ROWING FLAT BACK HINGE

ARM SPRINGS SET UP

- 2nd or 3rd eyebolt from the floor
- Adjust 1–2 eyebolts higher if you have a newer Springboard that goes up to 10 or 11

FUNCTIONS & TARGET MUSCLES

- Strengthens shoulder stabilizers and spinal erectors
- Works abdominals and stretches hamstrings
- Challenges memory, coordination, and control

ALIGNMENT CUES & OBSTACLES

- Really use abdominals to lengthen and stabilize spine
- Perform exercise with as much finesse and control as you can muster
- Lift slightly through sternum while hinging back and feel the chest open to the sky

ELLIE SAYS..."*The Springboard version of Flat Back Rowing is much simpler than the Reformer version...so enjoy!*"

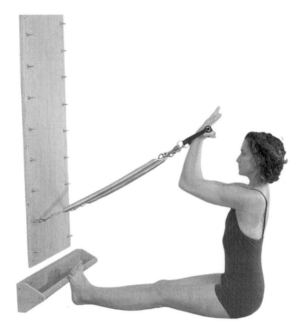

1. Starting Position — *3 repetitions*
Seated upright facing the Springboard, legs straight with feet flexed and in a Pilates "V". Arms are in front of the body with hands through handles. Elbows are bent to 90 degrees and even with the shoulders— "Pilates elbows." Palms face the body with fingers long.

Inhale and engage low glutes lifting torso up off the hips

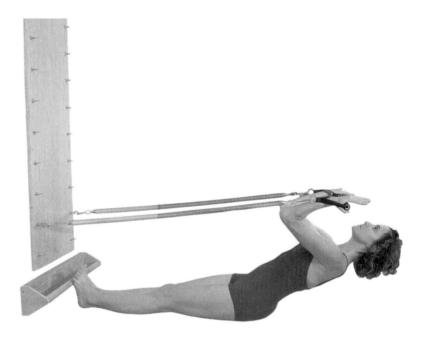

2. Exhale
Pull abdominals to spine and hinge backwards at hips, lifting chest slightly while performing a small bicep curl, keeping elbows high. Go back as far as you can maintain a stable spine.

3. Inhale and Exhale
Lift the chest and arms slightly as you return to the starting position, releasing bicep curl as you come forward.

CHEST EXPANSION

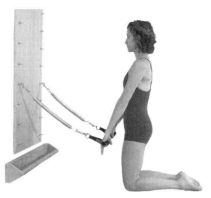

1. Starting Position — *4 repetitions*
Kneeling, hold the folded loops, pinkies facing back. Pitch forward slightly to engage hamstrings and glutes.

Inhale and lengthen spine

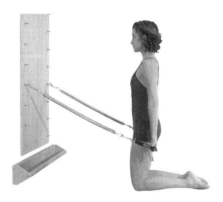

2. Exhale
Stabilize torso with abdominals, and pull arms back until even with sides (or a little further). Feel shoulders "smile" open.

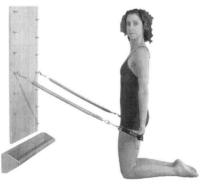

3–4. Inhale/Exhale
Look slowly from side to side, then look straight. Do not lean back or bend at hips while returning arms to starting position.

VARIATION: Rotator

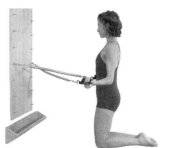

VARIATION: Rhomboids

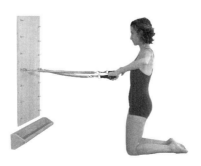

ARM SPRINGS SET UP
- 2nd–4th eyebolt from the floor
- Adjust 1–2 eyebolts higher if you have a newer Springboard that goes up to 10 or 11

FUNCTIONS & TARGET MUSCLES
- Strengthens lats, triceps, and rotator cuff
- Works hamstrings, glutes, and abdominals
- Challenges balance

ALIGNMENT CUES & OBSTACLES
- Do not crease at hips—really push femurs forward from the hamstrings to maintain one long line from knees to top of the head
- Focus on spine lengthening while moving arms—feel that invisible thread
- Keep neck relaxed and long—no forward head
- Place a rolled up pad under client's knees if kneeling causes any pain in patella
- **Obstacles:** Weak glutes, poor sense of balance
- **Contraindications:** Knee injuries, arthritis of the knees, sensitive knees

VARIATIONS & PEEL BACKS
- **Variation:** Also can be done with palms facing body for more rotator cuff action
- **Variations:** *Rotator*
  Hold handles with palms facing up. Keep elbows glued into body, and externally rotate arms, opening the shoulder. Repeat 5–8 times.
- **Variations:** *Rhomboids*
  Hold handles with palms facing down and pull elbows wide and back until you feel the mid-back working. Repeat 5–8 times.

IMAGINE... *you're a doll that your arms can move, but the back cannot, so you're hinging from your shoulder joint, not pulling with your pecs.*

ELLIE SAYS... *"Now this is really the 'perfect alignment' exercise."*

ARM CIRCLES

ARM SPRINGS SET UP

- 2nd–4th eyebolt from the floor
- Adjust 1–2 eyebolts higher if you have a newer Springboard that goes up to 10 or 11

FUNCTIONS & TARGET MUSCLES

- Strengthens deltoids and scapular stabilizers
- Works abdominals, glutes and hamstrings
- Challenges balance and control

ALIGNMENT CUES & OBSTACLES

- Really pitch forward as far as you can to work back of legs and to maximize the challenge of this exercise—feel the abdominals supporting the torso
- Warm up with 2–3 Queen arm reaches in this position before making full circles
- Keep arms in front of torso when opening arms and lowering them to sides
- Maintain even pressure of hands in loops through out the circle—use resistance to aid stabilization
- Move smoothly and with control—quick, jerking motions destabilize torso
- **Contraindication:** Some knee injuries (kneeling compresses the joint)

VARIATIONS & PEEL BACKS

- **Modifications:** *Offering*
  Begin with elbows by sides and forearms parallel to floor. Reach arms forward like you are offering a tray of margaritas to a party guest. Be sure not to lean back as you reach forward. Return arms to starting position.
- **Peel Backs:** *Kneeling Chest Expansion, Modified Front Rowing, Offering*

IMAGINE…you're being supported by a strong wind blowing against the front of your body—lean in to the wind.

ELLIE SAYS…"Press your heels like 'brakes' into stability bar to help stabilize."

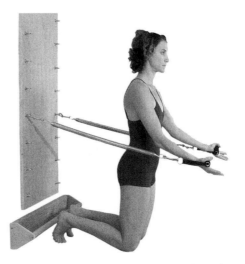

1. Starting Position — *3 repetitions in each direction*
Kneel with feet flexed and toes tucked under. Arms are by sides with hands through handles, palms facing up and wrists long.

Inhale to prepare

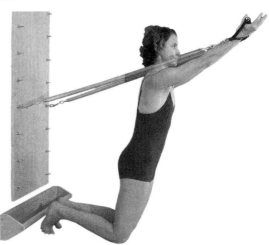

2. Exhale
Pull abdominals to spine, engage glutes and hamstrings, stabilize scapulae, and lift arms overhead (Queen reach). Keep palms facing up and feel scoop coming from scapulae.

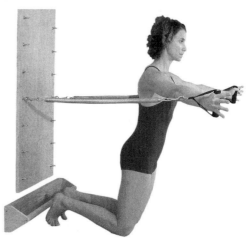

3. Exhale
Open arms out to sides with palms facing front and lower hands to sides returning to starting position. Maintain forward pitch of body while lowering the arms. Repeat twice more, and then reverse direction of circles. **Note:** When lowering arms in front of the body on reverse circle, palms should face up to facilitate open chest and stable scapulae.

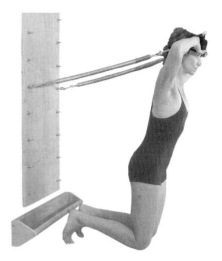

1. Starting Position — *4 repetitions*
Kneel with toes tucked under. Press heels into "stability bar" to engage hamstrings and glutes, and lean forward as far as you can. With hands in loops, salute forehead with elbows bent and index fingers touching eyebrows. Palms face out.

Inhale to prepare

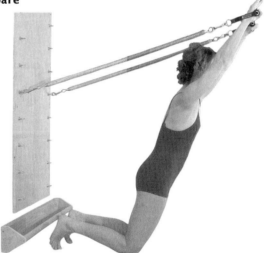

2–3. Exhale/Inhale
Pull abdominals to spine, push heels into stability bar to engage glutes and hamstrings, and stabilize scapulae while straightening elbows, keeping arms in line with body. Bend elbows and bring hands back to forehead while maintaining pitch of the body.

VARIATION: Shave Head

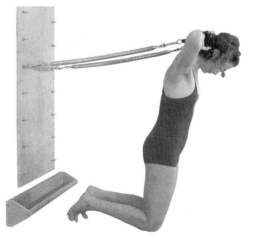

ARM SPRINGS SET UP
- 2nd–4th eyebolt from the floor
- Adjust 1–2 eyebolts higher if you have a newer Springboard that goes up to 10 or 11

FUNCTIONS & TARGET MUSCLES
- Strengthens triceps and deltoids
- Works abdominals, glutes, hamstrings, and mid traps
- Challenges balance and control

ALIGNMENT CUES & OBSTACLES
- Move smoothly and with control—quick, jerking motions destabilize torso
- Focus on the mid traps keeping scapulae stable
- Maintain pressure of arms in straps to stabilize when bending elbows
- **Obstacles:** Tight lats, weak glutes, fear of falling
- **Contraindication:** Some knee injuries (kneeling compresses the joint)

VARIATIONS & PEEL BACKS
- To decrease pressure on patellae, kneel upright, not pitched forward
- **Peel Back:** *Seated Salute*
- **Variation:** Shave off the back of the head for more challenge

IMAGINE...*you are a figurine carved into the prow of a ship and the entire ship supports you as you lean forward.*

ELLIE SAYS...*"Scary!"*

ARM SPRINGS SET UP

- Handles attached, at the level of your shoulders

FUNCTIONS & TARGET MUSCLES

- Strengthens triceps and legs
- Trains shoulder stability
- Teaches you how to punch

ALIGNMENT CUES & OBSTACLES

- The standing arm springs exercises comprise a wonderful full body stabilization and conditioning series. *Punching* is the only exercise in this series done in a lunge. The rest will be done in a forward pitch. See *Hug A Tree* for details.

- As you punch, don't let the shoulder roll forward; stabilize the shoulder blade with your back and shoulder muscles

- **Variations:** In the lunging position, you can do *Hug A Tree, Salute*

IMAGINE...*you are Rocky—in the first movie, of course.*

ELLIE SAYS...*"Feeling strong now!"*

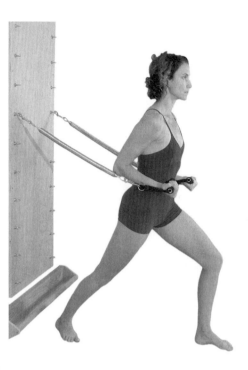

1. Starting Position — *8 punches alternating arms, then repeat with other leg forward in lunge*

Stand in a lunge facing away from the Springboard with your back heel lifted and pressing into the foot bar to support the back leg. Holding the handles with fists facing up then bend elbows to your sides.

Inhale to prepare

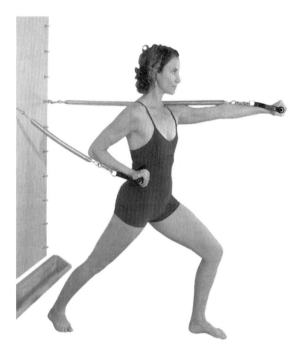

2. Exhale

Punch one arm forward, turning the fist downward as you aim straight ahead, keeping fist in line with your shoulder.

Come back to the starting position and alternate sides. After 8 punches, bring the other leg forward into the lunge.

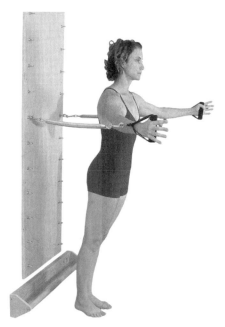

1. Starting Position — *6 repetitions*

Stand with your back to Springboard with feet close to the foot bar, in Pilates "V" or Parallel. Place your hands in the handles with arms to sides with hands and elbows slightly lower than shoulders. Elbows are slightly rounded. Arms are slightly in front of torso. You should be able to see your elbows in your peripheral vision. These are "ballet arms." Pitch your whole body forward so that you are a diagonal line from feet to head, leaning into the resistance.

Inhale and scoop the belly in, lengthen spine, squeeze inner thighs and glutes

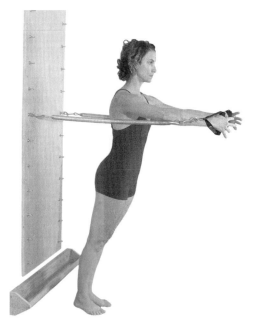

2. Exhale

Keeping back wide and spine long, pull hands toward one another as if you were hugging a tree. Keep elbows rounded.

3. Inhale

Open arms to starting position, maintaining pitch of body.

After 3 repetitions reverse the breathing so the arms pull together on inhale for 3 more repetitions. Breathe into the lateral ribs as you initiate the hug.

ARM SPRINGS SET UP

- Handles attached, at the level of your shoulders

FUNCTIONS & TARGET MUSCLES

- Strengthens deltoids and pec major
- Works abdominals, inner thighs, glutes
- Teaches scapular stabilization with humeral motion (mid trap, serratus anterior, rhomboids)

ALIGNMENT CUES & OBSTACLES

- Make sure to flow through the following four exercises: *Hug A Tree, Salute, Full Arm Circles* and *Butterfly,* maintaining your forward pitch the whole time to maximize the work of the glutes, hamstrings, inner thighs and abdominals. The standing arm springs series is a great option for people who cannot kneel.
- Keep head aligned over pelvis in excellent standing posture while moving arms
- Sit right on sits bones—no slouching behind them or arching in front of them
- Feel chest and back staying wide and stable as arms move
- Reach through pinky finger to encourage the serratus anterior to work
- As arms return to starting position, do not let elbows move behind torso—this will pinch shoulder blades and force pecs to initiate the next "hug"
- Think "ballet arms"

IMAGINE...*you're a doll and your arms can move, but the back cannot, so you're hinging from your shoulder joint, not pulling with your pecs.*

ELLIE SAYS...*"Romana used to call this Hug Pavarotti."*

SALUTE

ARM SPRINGS SET UP

- Handles attached, at the level of your shoulders

FUNCTIONS & TARGET MUSCLES

- Strengthens triceps and deltoids
- Works abdominals, inner thighs, and glutes
- Teaches shoulder girdle stability

ALIGNMENT CUES & OBSTACLES

- Transition directly from Hug A Tree, maintaining your forward pitch.
- Keep shoulders wide and scapula sliding down back—DO NOT OVERUSE UPPER TRAPS (it is very difficult to not overuse upper traps and levator scapula)
- If it is difficult to keep shoulders down, allow arms to widen as they extend— saluting more toward the side than the front
- **Obstacles:** Tight upper traps, tight lats carpal tunnel and upper quarter Repetitive Stress Injury issues

VARIATIONS & PEEL BACKS

- **Modification:** Widen arms on extension if client has tight shoulders.
- **Peel Backs:** *Double Lat Pulls* on the Cadillac (both versions), seated *Salute* on Reformer or Springboard

IMAGINE…you are saluting the Pilates Goddess.

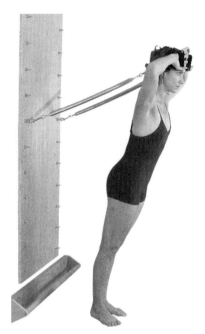

1. Starting Position — *6 repetitions*
From your last repetition of *Hug A Tree* (arms open to the sides with soft elbows), straighten your arms diagonally forward, shoulder distance apart, still leaning into the resistance and maintain your forward pitch. Then *Salute* forehead by bending elbows, index fingers touching eyebrows with palms facing out.

Inhale to prepare

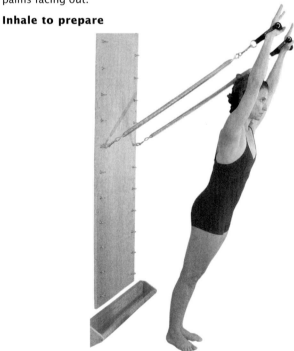

2. Exhale
Straighten elbows while stabilizing scapulae so they don't elevate. Arms straighten to doorframe position on the line of the body. Hands are even with or wider than shoulders.

3. Inhale
Elbows bend and fingers return to eyebrows. Repeat 3 times.

4. Exhale
Drop head forward bringing hands behind head and *Salute* the Pilates Goddess from this position (like you're shaving off the back of your head).

5. Inhale
Return to starting position with control.

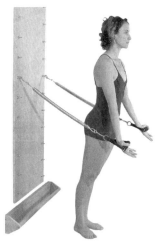

1. Starting Position — *6 repetitions*
From the last *Salute* (arms extended diagonally forward and up, shoulder distance apart), open your arms slowly to your sides, softening the elbows, as if you are stroking a huge globe in front of you. Keep leaning into the resistance and maintain your forward pitch as your arms circle down to your hips, ending with palms facing up.

Inhale to prepare

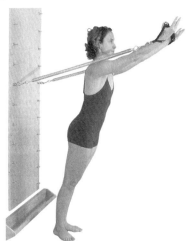

2. Exhale
Feel the shoulder blades dropping down the back as you bring your arms up in front of you, shoulder distance apart, elbows soft, until they are up as high as you can reach without your shoulders rising.

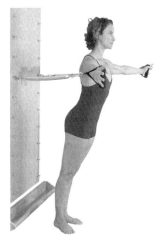

3. Inhale
Turn your palms forward slowly as you transition into the arm circling out to the sides, again stroking a huge globe in front of you.

Repeat 3 times and switch directions.

ARM SPRINGS SET UP
- Handles attached, at the level of your shoulders

FUNCTIONS & TARGET MUSCLES
- Strengthens pectorals, biceps, and serratus anterior
- Works abdominals, inner thighs, glutes
- Teaches shoulder girdle stability

ALIGNMENT CUES & OBSTACLES
- Transition into *Circles* directly from *Salute* and maintain your forward pitch
- Keep shoulders wide and scapula sliding down back—DO NOT OVERUSE UPPER TRAPS
- **Obstacles:** Tight upper traps, tight lats carpal tunnel and upper quarter RSI issues

VARIATIONS & PEEL BACKS
- **Modification:** Widen arms on extension if client has tight shoulders
- **Peel Backs:** *Double Lat Pulls* on the Cadillac (both versions), *Hug a Tree* on the Reformer or Springboard with arm springs either seated or standing

IMAGINE...*you are stroking a globe in front of you.*

ELLIE SAYS...*"Wow, this one really challenges core stability. Really try to keep your forward pitch through the whole circle!"*

ARM SPRINGS SET UP

- Handles attached, at the level of your shoulders

FUNCTIONS & TARGET MUSCLES

- Trains scapular stability; specifically the balance between the rhomboids/mid traps and serratus anterior
- Strengthens the pecs, glutes, hamstrings, inner thighs and abdominals

ALIGNMENT CUES & OBSTACLES

- Transition into *Butterfly* from *Full Arm Circles* and maintain your forward pitch
- Keep shoulder blades perfectly stable as you open and close the arms
- Don't let arms open too wide so that they are behind your torso

VARIATIONS & PEEL BACKS

- **Peel Back:** *Hug a Tree*

IMAGINE...*you are a butterfly in the mountains.*

ELLIE SAYS...*"This is one of the best shoulder stabilization exercises around."*

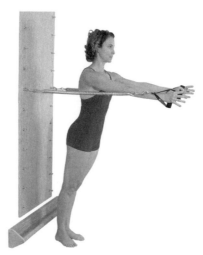

1. Starting Position — *4 times alternating arms, 4 times both arms*
Transition from *Full Arm Circles* (arms down by your hips with soft elbows), by straightening your elbows and reaching arms forward until they are shoulder height and shoulder distance apart, as if you are standing on your arms in a plank position, but with palms facing each other.

Inhale to prepare

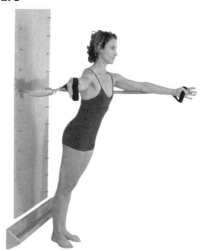

2. Exhale
Slowly open one arm to the side, keeping it at shoulder height.

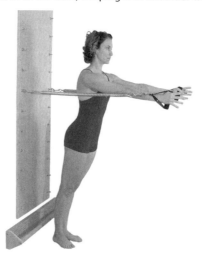

3. Inhale (and Exhale and Inhale)
Return to starting position and alternate sides 4 times.

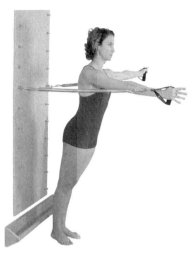

4. Exhale
Slowly open both arms to the sides, like a butterfly.

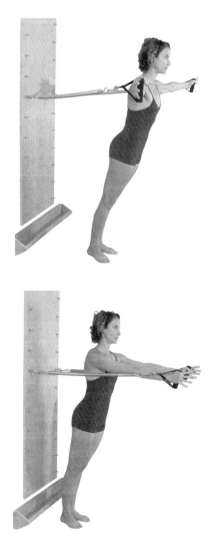

5. Inhale
Return to starting position. Repeat full Butterfly 3–7 more times.

ARM SPRINGS SET UP

- 7th–9th eyebolt from the floor depending on height of person
- Adjust 1–2 eyebolts higher if you have a newer Springboard that goes up to 10 or 11

FUNCTIONS & TARGET MUSCLES

- Strengthens quads, hamstrings, glutes and biceps

ALIGNMENT CUES & OBSTACLES

- Keep your knees aiming over your 3rd toes
- Keep the shoulders open and shoulder blades pulling down the back

VARIATIONS & PEEL BACKS

- **Variation:** (not shown) *Squat with knees and feet together* (Utkatasana in yoga). Try the squat keeping knees and feet squeezing together, and bend knees to a 90 degree angle, leaning slightly forward from torso. Allow pelvis to be neutral or even slightly in anterior tilt (stick your butt out a little) and then pull up from the pelvic floor and low belly to lengthen low back. Hold for 10–30 seconds or add arm pulls below.
- **See opposite page**

IMAGINE...*you are sitting down on an invisible chair.*

ELLIE SAYS...*"Great for the bootay."*

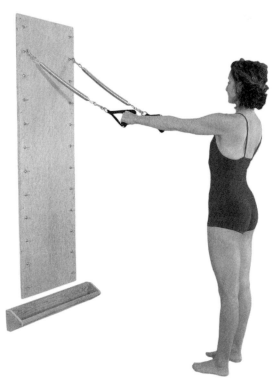

1. Starting Position — *8 repetitions*
Stand facing the Springboard, with legs hip distance apart, holding the handles with arms extended. Your arms should be pulling into the resistance.

Inhale to prepare

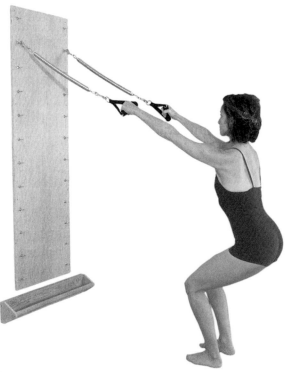

2. Exhale
Press into your heels and bend your knees, coming down into a squat, no lower than 90 degree angle at your knees. Stick your butt out a little.

VARIATION: Squat with arm double pulls

Hold for 10–30 seconds then come back up or add arm pulls.

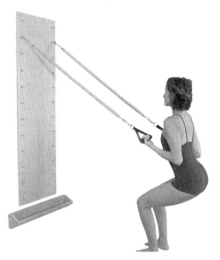

VARIATION: Alternating Single Arm Pulls

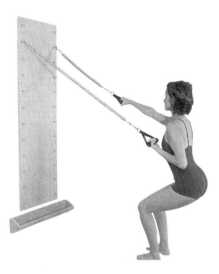

VARIATION: Squat in 2nd Position

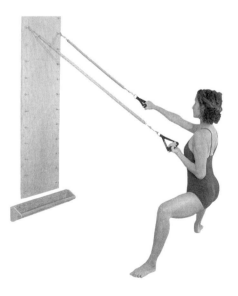

VARIATIONS & PEEL BACKS

- **Variation:** *Squat with Arm Pulls:* Try either squat and add 8 arm pulls, pulling elbows wide to the sides while holding your squat, allowing fists to rotate so palm turns up as you pull it in to the side of your body. Then try alternating arm pulls, allowing each arm to complete the full movement before alternating. Keep shoulders stabilized as spring pulls arm forward; don't allow humerus to roll forward.

- **Variation:** *Squat* in 2nd position: Legs open wide and turned out

3-WAY PECTORAL STRETCH *standing arm springs series*

ARM SPRINGS SET UP

- Handles attached, the highest eyebolt up as you can reach

FUNCTIONS & TARGET MUSCLES

- Stretches the chest and pectoral muscles
- Activates the upper back muscles

ALIGNMENT CUES & OBSTACLES

- Stick your chest out and lean into the stretch
- Take deep inhales and allow the spaces between the ribs (the intercostals) to expand and stretch
- The *3-Way Pec Stretch* is a great finish to the standing arm series

IMAGINE...you are Kate Winslet suspended off the front of the Titanic.

ELLIE SAYS..."This is a great stretch to do at the end of a session to feel the chest opening."

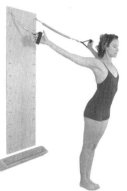

1. Starting Position — *1 set*
Stand facing away from the Springboard, holding the arm springs behind you. Begin with your arms diagonally reaching back above your head (making a "V" shape) elbows facing each other, palms facing away from each other. Open your arms against the resistance.
Exhale
Pull the arms closer together behind you. Hold for one full breath, allow the chest to expand and open forward. Think of squeezing the scapulae together behind you.

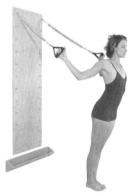

2. Inhale
Open your arms against the resistance and lower them so that they are in line with your armpits making a "T" shape, with arms behind the torso and bend your elbows to increase the stretch.
Exhale
Pull the arms closer together behind you. Hold for one full breath, allowing the chest to expand and open forward. Think of squeezing the scapulae together behind you.

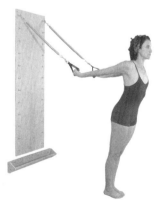

3. Inhale
Open your arms against the resistance and lower them slightly, then internally rotate the arms, turning the elbows out and the palms toward each other.
Exhale
Pull the arms closer together behind you. Hold for one full breath, allowing the chest to expand and open forward. Think of squeezing the scapulae together behind you.

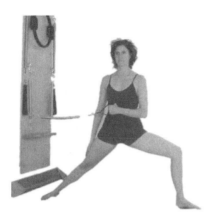

1. Starting Position — *4 or 5 times each side*
Stand with your side to the springboard, holding the arm handle in your outside hand, elbow bent, and glued to the side of your torso. Come into in a yoga "Warrior 2" position with your legs: your straight leg parallel with your foot close to the springboard and facing forward, your lunging leg externally rotated, foot turned out, knee bent at a ninety degree angle, femur externally rotated so that the knee aims over the third toe.

Inhale to prepare

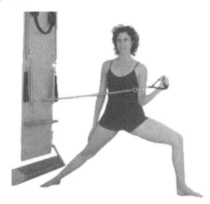

2. Exhale
Externally rotate the working arm, keeping the elbow glued to the side of your torso.

3. Inhale
Hold for a moment, making sure to completely rotate the head of the humerus and really feel the scapula anchoring into the back; connecting to the rhomboids.

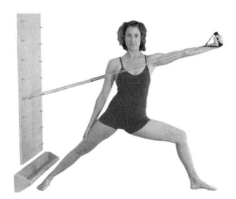

4. Exhale
Extend the arm diagonally to the side, like you are punching something sideways, at the height of your shoulder.

5. Inhale/Exhale
Retrograde the movement and return to the starting position.

ARM SPRINGS SET UP
- 2nd or 3rd eyebolt from the floor
- Adjust 1–2 eyebolts higher if you have a newer Springboard that goes up to 10 or 11

FUNCTIONS & TARGET MUSCLES
- Strengthens the rotator cuff
- Teaches stabilization of the shoulder through connecting the scapula to the back
- Strengthens the quads, glutes, hamstrings

ALIGNMENT CUES & OBSTACLES
- Keep lunging knee aimed over 3rd toe

IMAGINE...*you are a warrior goddess.*

ELLIE SAYS...*"This is one of the best shoulder stabilization exercises around."*

SWACKADEE

ARM SPRINGS SET UP

- 2nd or 3rd eyebolt from the floor
- Adjust 1–2 eyebolts higher if you have a newer Springboard that goes up to 10 or 11

FUNCTIONS & TARGET MUSCLES

- Strengthens the shoulder girdle and wrist
- Great for tennis players
- Strengthens the quads, glutes, hamstrings

ALIGNMENT CUES & OBSTACLES

- Keep lunging knee aimed over 3rd toe
- Think: elbow, wrist, hand
- Keep wrist long and strong

IMAGINE...*you are a warrior goddess.*

ELLIE SAYS...*"Do this exercise with flow and momentum or else you'll load the wrist too much."*

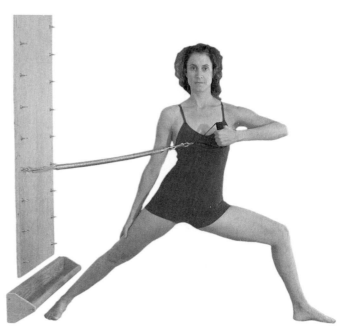

1. Starting Position — *4 or 5 times each side*
Stand with your side to the Springboard, holding the arm handle in your outside hand, elbow bent, forearm in front of your torso. Come into in a yoga "Warrior 2" position with your legs: your straight leg parallel with your foot close to the springboard and facing forward, your lunging leg externally rotated, foot turned out, knee bent at a 90 degree angle, femur externally rotated so that the knee aims over the 3rd toe.

Inhale to prepare

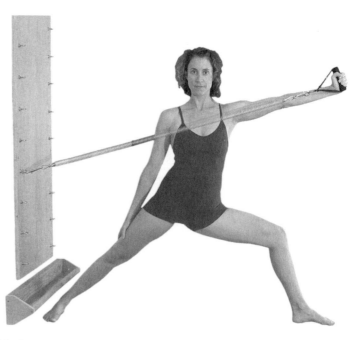

2. Exhale
Extend your arm diagonally to the side, as if you are pulling a long sword from your belt and raising it to the opposite side.

3. Inhale (and Exhale and Inhale)
Return to starting position.

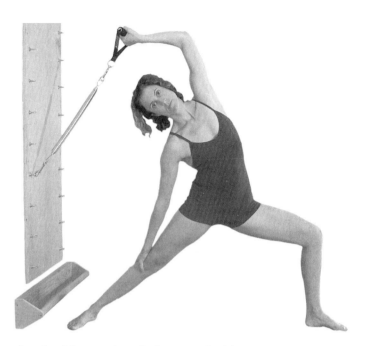

1. Starting Position — *4 or 5 times each side*

Stand with your side to the springboard and come into in a "Warrior 2" position with your legs: your straight leg parallel with your foot close to the springboard and facing forward, your lunging leg externally rotated, foot turned out, knee bent at a 90 degree angle, femur externally rotated so that the knee aims over the third toe. Hold the arm handle in your outside hand and side bend your torso toward the springboard, lifting your elbow so that it points toward the sky, palm facing up, and supporting your body with the other arm on your bent knee.

Inhale to prepare

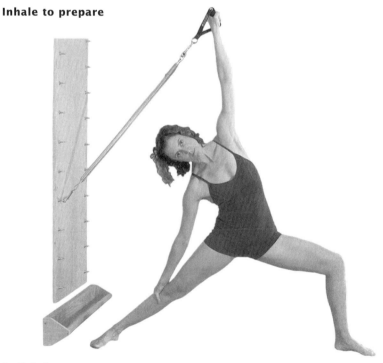

2. Exhale

Keep your shoulder fixed and anchored down into the back and away from the head, extend your elbow so that your hand reaches up to the sky.

3. Inhale (and Exhale and Inhale)

Return to starting position.

ARM SPRINGS SET UP

- 2nd or 3rd eyebolt from the floor
- Adjust 1–2 eyebolts higher if you have a newer Springboard that goes up to 10 or 11

FUNCTIONS & TARGET MUSCLES

- Stretches the lats, obliques and QL's
- Strengthens the shoulder girdle
- Strengthens the quads, glutes, hamstrings

ALIGNMENT CUES & OBSTACLES

- Keep lunging knee aimed over 3rd toe
- Your elbow should stay absolutely stable as you extend and bend the working arm
- Keep the neck long by keeping the shoulder glued down into the back
- **Contraindication:** Unstable shoulders

VARIATIONS & PEEL BACKS

- Try a set with palm facing down

IMAGINE...you are a warrior goddess painting under the stairs.

ELLIE SAYS..."Do this exercise with flow and momentum or else you'll load the wrist too much."

ARM SPRINGS SET UP
- 2nd or 3rd eyebolt from the floor
- Adjust 1–2 eyebolts higher if you have a newer Springboard that goes up to 10 or 11

FUNCTIONS & TARGET MUSCLES
- Challenges coordination and balance
- Trains stabilization of the shoulder girdle
- Strengthens the pectorals, quads, glutes, hamstrings

ALIGNMENT CUES & OBSTACLES
- Keep lunging knee aimed over 3rd toe
- Keep body stable, using obliques to keep torso from twisting
- Keep shoulders down away from ears
- On return movement, be sure to keep scapulae wide in the back; do not let them squeeze together, thus balancing the work of the serratus anterior and rhomboids

VARIATIONS & PEEL BACKS
- **Peel Back:** Seated and standing *Hug a Tree.*

IMAGINE... *you have a resistance in both arms.*

ELLIE SAYS... *"I made this one up to throw a little asymmetry into the series."*

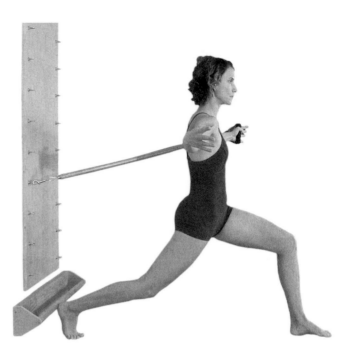

1. Starting Position — *4 or 5 times each side*
Transition from *Lunging Painting Under the Stairs* by rotating body and legs to face away from Springboard, coming under the working arm (which holds the arm spring), and bringing both arms out to the side, in a ballet "second position," with soft elbows and palms facing forward. This is the classic starting arm position for *Hug A Tree,* but only one arm is in the spring, and the spring should be coming from the far eyebolt, crossing diagonally behind your back.

Inhale to prepare

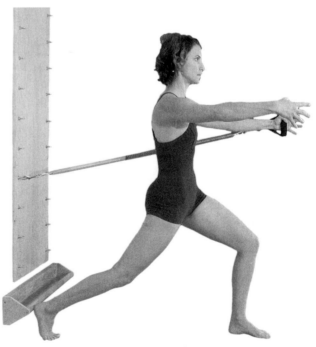

2. Exhale
Hug a tree. A huge tree; a sequoia, a redwood. Hug arotti. Use obliques to stabilize torso

3. Inhale
Return to starting position.

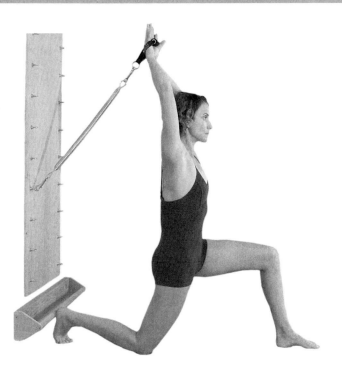

1. Starting Position — *3 times each side*
Transition from *One Arm Hug a Tree* by coming down into a kneeling lunge, bringing your back knee onto the floor, and slip both hands into the arm handle as you bring the handle above your head.

Inhale to prepare

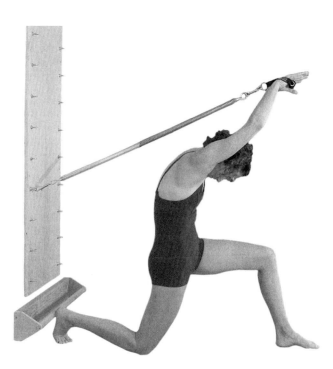

2. Exhale
Tuck your pelvis under by scooping in your belly and squeezing your glutes as you arc your arms and upper body forward (like a cobra rearing its head). Allow your head to come forward and down, bringing your upper spine into flexion until you feel a deep psoas stretch, deep in the lower back.

3. Inhale (and Exhale and Inhale)
Return to starting position and repeat 3 times.

ARM SPRINGS SET UP
- 2nd or 3rd eyebolt from the floor
- Adjust 1–2 eyebolts higher if you have a newer Springboard that goes up to 10 or 11

FUNCTIONS & TARGET MUSCLES
- Stretches psoas and other hip flexors

ALIGNMENT CUES & OBSTACLES
- Try hissing while you do this. It helps to find your inner cobra
- Keep your center over your knee—only your head, neck, and thoracic spine round forward

IMAGINE...*you are a cobra rearing its angry head.*

ELLIE SAYS... *"We call this a 'dural' stretch for the psoas because it stretches the lumbar spine attachments of the psoas. The 'dura mater' is the covering of the spinal cord. Thus you should feel this particular stretch deep in the back... not just the front of the hip."*

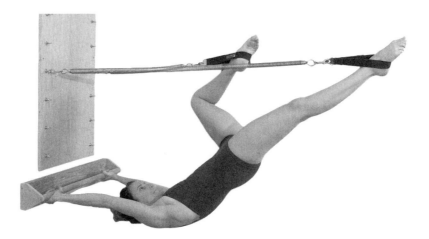

With all the leg spring exercises, the motion of the legs works the hamstrings and adductors while challenging the stability of the pelvis and spine. Work within a range of motion that allows for stability. As strength and stability increase, so will the range of motion.

WHERE TO PLACE THE LEG SPRINGS:

The height at which to attach the springs will vary according to the strength of the springs and the weight of the person. You should be able to pull the springs with your legs without losing core stability and without sliding back toward the springboard. For very petite people, you may need to put a sticky pad under your torso to keep from sliding.

LEG SPRINGS: BREAKDOWN OF LEVELS

Fundamental

Single Leg Springs is a great way to start teaching the concept of moving the leg independently of the pelvis. Also it's great for people with lower limb injuries or for the more motor-challenged individuals. Working one leg at a time trains contra-lateral pelvic stabilization; i.e. it works the obliques. Start by lying with one spring aligned with the hip of the working leg.

Beginning /Intermediate

Double Leg Springs is a great way to strengthen the legs while teaching neutral pelvis and training pelvic stability. If client is unable maintain a stable pelvis, do the *Single Leg Series* instead. These exercises are excellent for spine, knee and hip rehabilitation.

Side Leg Springs can be a very challenging core stabilization series. Modeled after the *Side Kick Series* on the mat, *Side Leg Springs* work the gluteus medius, gluteus maximus and the adductors. Great for pregnant clients throughout their pregnancy.

Super Advanced

Magician Series is basically the *Double Leg Springs* done in levitation. In order to accomplish this you must increase the resistance by quite a lot. Normally you would raise the height of the springs by two-fold. This series can be very loaded on the neck, so don't do with neck-sensitive clients. Only attempt when client has an extreme amount of core strength. *The Dolphin* with levitation and *Diamond Pulls* with levitation are good exercises to start with because you don't have to maintain levitation for a prolonged period of time. Once someone can hold their body in a complete and perfect plank in their Dolphin, then you can start adding on more exercises into the *Magician Series*. The turned-out variations are much easier to levitate because the Powerhouse is more accessible in external rotation (inner thighs and glute max are engaged). When selecting which exercises to do keep this in mind. Don't try to do all the exercises in a row at first; start with less and rest in between or do the Dolphin as a semi-resting transition. Start by raising the springs 2–4 eyebolts and really press yourself away from the foot bar by extending long through the arms.

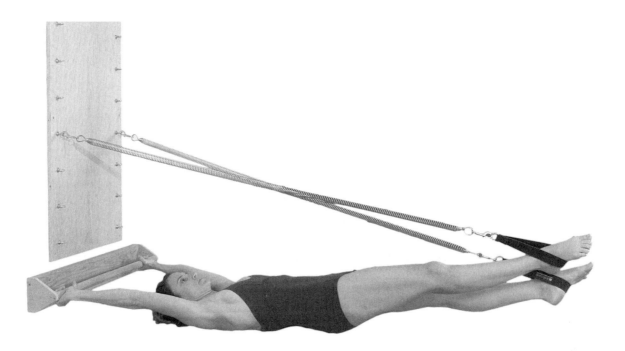

GENERAL ALIGNMENT CUES FOR ALL SUPINE LEG SERIES

• Do not initiate "pull" with back muscles—maintain neutral pelvis and spine

• Keep ROM small and monitor client's neutral spine with a hand under the lumbar spine

• When working in parallel, keep knees bent 1 to 2 degrees to avoid locking and/or hyperextending knee

• Initiate pull from the top of the femur, not the feet—focus on medial hamstring

• (For posterior pelvis)—To avoid tucking pelvis, think of the pubic bone rotating down while legs return to starting position

• (For anterior pelvis)—Focus on the top of the sacrum staying connected to mat as legs pull down—the end range of the movement is just before sacrum destabilizes

• Normal hamstring flexibility is hip flexion to 80 degrees, so most clients will not be able to perform this exercise in the prescribed ROM of 90 degrees to 35 degrees of hip flexion

• Feel legs lengthen away from torso as torso lengthens away from legs (opposing energy helps to create stability)

• Place hand under client's lumbar spine to monitor neutral pelvis and spine extensors, and/or place hand on low abdominals to monitor client's scoop

• Keep feet relaxed—neither pointed nor flexed

• Contraindications: Acute phase of hamstring pull, strain, or tear

GENERAL MODIFICATIONS, VARIATIONS AND PEEL BACKS

Modifications: If client is small or finds maintaining neutral difficult, lighten the resistance.
If there is neck strain, arms can be down by your side instead of holding onto the bar

Variation: To focus on pelvic stability, use thigh straps (or loops) placed above the knees (as opposed to on the feet) to create a smaller ROM

Peel Back: *Single Leg Spring* exercises are easier than double leg springs, so you can always start with them, especially with people who have difficulty maintaining pelvis stability and neutral spine

LEG SPRINGS SET UP

- 2nd–4th eyebolt from the floor
- Adjust 1–2 eyebolts higher if you have a newer Springboard that goes up to 10 or 11

FUNCTIONS & TARGET MUSCLES

- Strengthens hamstrings
- Teaches pelvic stability while the legs move up and down
- Teaches disassociation of the femur from the pelvis
- Single Leg work teaches contralateral stabilization, working the obliques

ALIGNMENT CUES & OBSTACLES

- See Leg Springs General Alignment Cues
- Straighten non-working leg if client's hamstrings are not too tight

VARIATIONS & PEEL BACKS

- **Modification:** If client is small or finds maintaining neutral difficult, use lighter resistance
- **Variation:** To focus on pelvic stability, use thigh straps (or loops) placed above the knees (as opposed to on the feet) to create a smaller ROM

IMAGINE..._your leg is not attached to your body, but moves freely up and down._

ELLIE SAYS..._"This is a great way to teach the separation of the leg from the torso."_

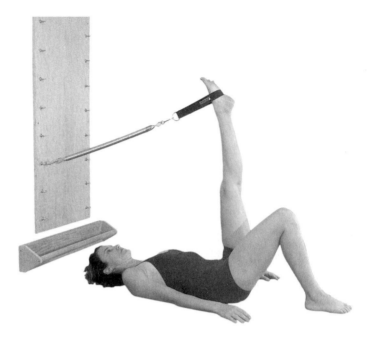

1. Starting Position — *4 to 6 repetitions in each direction*
Supine with one knee bent with foot on the mat and the other foot in the cotton loop, leg extended parallel and as high as possible without losing neutral pelvis.

Inhale to prepare

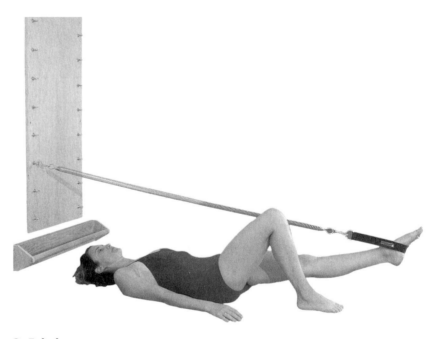

2. Exhale
Engage abdominal scoop and pull leg down as far as possible without losing abdominal scoop.

3. Inhale
Control the leg back up to the starting position.

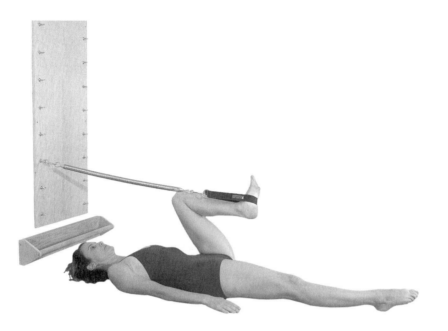

LEG SPRINGS SET UP

- 2nd–4th eyebolt from the floor
- Adjust 1–2 eyebolts higher if you have a newer Springboard that goes up to 10 or 11

FUNCTIONS & TARGET MUSCLES

- Single Leg work teaches contralateral stabilization, working the obliques

ALIGNMENT CUES & OBSTACLES

- See Leg Springs General Alignment Cues
- Keep knee just outside spring
- Use obliques to stabilize pelvis

VARIATIONS & PEEL BACKS

- **Modification:** If client has tight hamstrings, and is unable to maintain neutral pelvis with leg long on the mat, bend the non-working leg and place the foot on the mat

IMAGINE...*your pelvis is nailed down on the non-working side.*

ELLIE SAYS...*"This is a great way to introduce pelvic stabilization."*

1. Starting Position — *4 to 8 repetitions in each position*
Supine with one leg long on the mat and the other foot in the cotton loop with knee bent in a frog squat; hip externally rotated just enough that the knee clears the outside of the spring.

Inhale to prepare

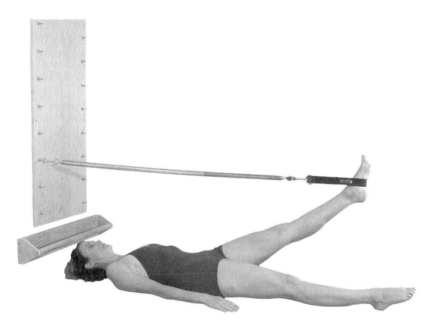

2. Exhale
Engage abdominal scoop and extend bent leg, pressing heel long away from you, keeping leg at about a 45 degree angle from the floor.

3. Inhale
Control back to starting position without tucking pelvis. Ground the coccyx into mat.

SINGLE LEG OVALS

LEG SPRINGS SET UP

- 2nd–4th eyebolt from the floor
- Adjust 1–2 eyebolts higher if you have a newer Springboard that goes up to 10 or 11

FUNCTIONS & TARGET MUSCLES

- Trains full ROM of hip joint; external and internal rotation
- Strengthens hamstrings
- Teaches pelvic stability while the legs move up and down
- Teaches disassociation of the femur from the pelvis
- Single leg work teaches contralateral stabilization, working the obliques

ALIGNMENT CUES & OBSTACLES

- See Leg Springs General Alignment Cues

VARIATIONS & PEEL BACKS

- **Modification:** If client has tight hamstrings, and is unable to maintain neutral pelvis with leg long on the mat, bend the non-working leg and place the foot on the mat

IMAGINE...*you are juicing up the acetabulum.*

ELLIE SAYS...*"This is a great way to lubricate the hip joint."*

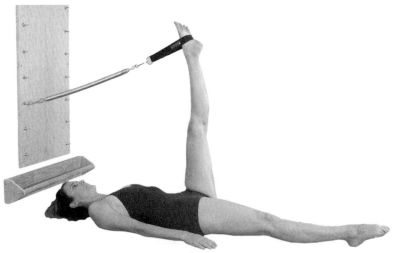

1. Starting Position — *4 to 6 repetitions in each direction*

Supine with one leg long on the mat and the other foot in the cotton loop, leg extended and as high as possible without losing neutral pelvis.

Inhale to prepare

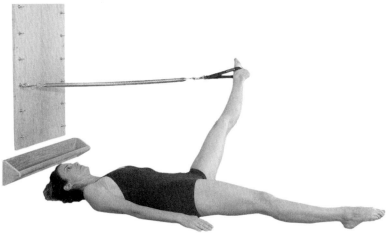

2. Exhale

Engage abdominal scoop and externally rotate working hip as you draw an oval with your heel. Open to the side first, then pull down as far as possible without loosing abdominal scoop.

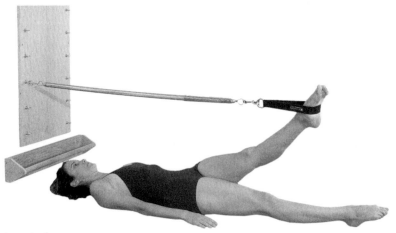

3. Inhale

Continue the oval by allowing working leg to internally rotate as it crosses over the center line and back up to the starting position.

Repeat 3–6 times and reverse directions.

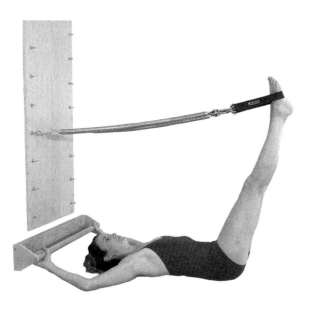

1. Starting Position — *4 to 8 repetitions in each position*
Straps around arches of feet, legs parallel with heels in line with sits bones, spine is neutral with hips in flexion. Knees are ever so softly bent.

Inhale to prepare

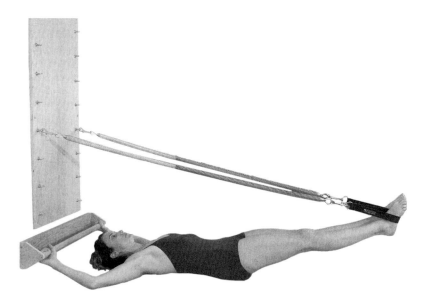

2. Exhale
Engage abdominal scoop and pull legs down toward mat without losing neutral pelvis/spine. Focus on top of sacrum staying connected to mat.

3. Inhale
Control legs back to starting position without tucking pelvis. Ground the coccyx into mat using low abdominals.

LEG SPRINGS SET UP
- 2nd–4th eyebolt from the floor
- Adjust 1–2 eyebolts higher if you have a newer Springboard that goes up to 10 or 11

FUNCTIONS & TARGET MUSCLES
- Teaches pelvic stability while the legs move up and down
- Hamstrings pull legs toward mat, and adductors keep legs parallel or together when hips are in turned out position
- Teaches disassociation of the femur from the pelvis

ALIGNMENT CUES & OBSTACLES
- See Leg Springs General Alignment Cues

VARIATIONS & PEEL BACKS
- **Variation:** To work adductors more keep ankles, knees, and thighs touching
- **Peel Back:** *Single Leg Spring Pulls*

IMAGINE... Barbie's pelvis and legs—there is no way for her pelvis to move with her legs.

SUSI SAYS..."When I first learned this exercise I could only move my legs in about in a 20 degree ROM without overusing my back extensors. So don't be afraid to work small."

VARIATION: Turned Out — *4 to 8 repetitions*
Rotate hip externally so feet are in Pilates "V"—keep heels together and knees straight (if heels are together knee joint cannot hyperextend).

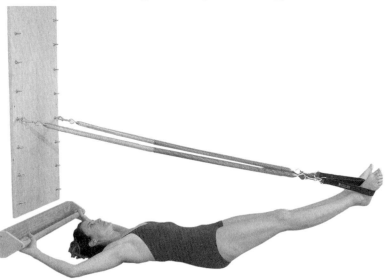

VARIATION: Turned In — *4 to 8 repetitions*
Start with legs in parallel, heels in line with sits bones, internally rotate femurs until toes touch (do not turn in at ankle joint).

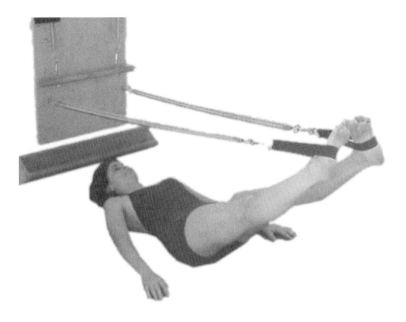

VARIATION: Running

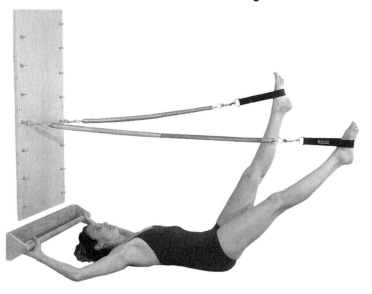

- **Variation:** *Running in Parallel:*
  Start with both legs up and in parallel and pull legs alternately down toward the floor in small pulses, controlling the springs so there is no rebound movement. Running down 2,3,4,5,6,7,8 and up 2,3,4,5,6,7,8

- **Variation:** *Scissors in Turn Out:*
  Start with both legs up turned-out and scissor legs in small movements crossing one foot on top of the other, alternately down toward the floor in small pulses, controlling the springs so there is no rebound movement. Scissor down 2,3,4,5,6,7,8 and up 2,3,4,5,6,7,8.

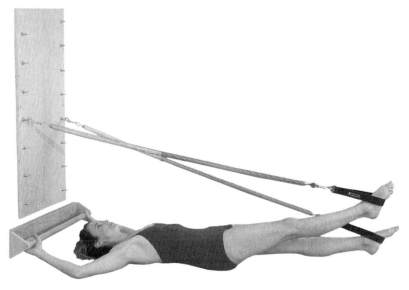

VARIATION: Scissors

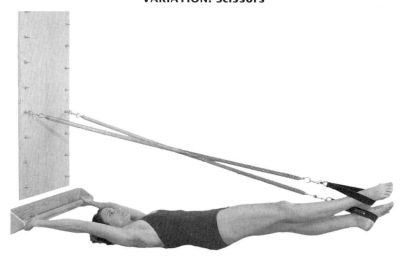

LEG SPRINGS SET UP

- 2nd–4th eyebolt from the floor
- Adjust 1–2 eyebolts higher if you have a newer Springboard that goes up to 10 or 11

FUNCTIONS & TARGET MUSCLES

- Strengthens hamstrings and adductors
- Abdominals and deep spinal muscles stabilize pelvis and spine while hip moves through wide ROM
- Teaches disassociation of the femur from the pelvis as hips move in multiple planes

ALIGNMENT CUES & OBSTACLES

- Focus on moving from the top of the femur—closer to the body's center than the feet
- Keep movement precise and really differentiate

VARIATIONS & PEEL BACKS

- **Peel Backs:** *Leg Pulls* and *Open/Close*

IMAGINE...*your feet are the lead point of a pencil and you are drawing rectangles in the air.*

ELLIE SAYS...*"No abdominal pooching when you lower or open your legs!"*

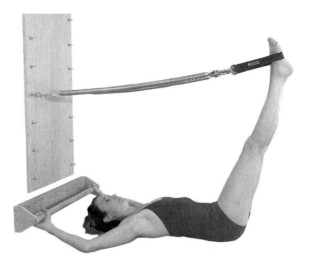

1. Starting Position — *4 repetitions in each direction*
Straps around arches of feet, legs parallel with inner thighs squeezing together. Spine is neutral. Knees ever so softly bent.

Inhale to prepare

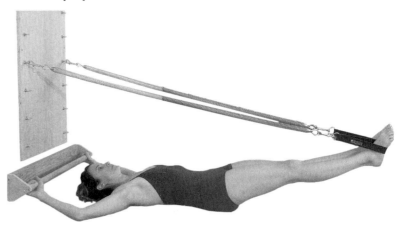

2. Exhale
Feel abdominals pull to spine keeping pelvis neutral, and pull legs down through the center and open hip distance apart.

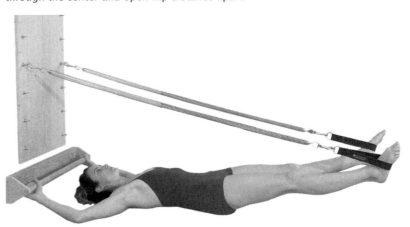

3. Open legs hip distance apart.

4. Inhale
Raise legs, then close them to starting position without losing neutral.

Repeat 4 times then reverse directions

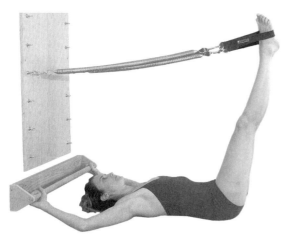

1. Starting Position — *4 repetitions in each direction*

Straps around arches of feet, rotate hips externally so feet are in Pilates "V." For Turned In: Start with legs in parallel, heels in line with sits bones, internally rotate femurs until toes touch (do not turn in at ankle joint).

Inhale to prepare

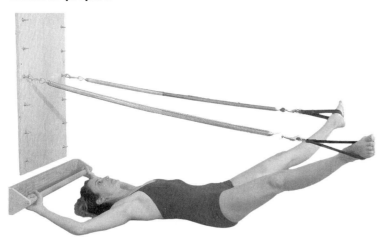

2. Exhale

Feel abdominals pull to spine, keeping pelvis neutral, and circle legs open a little wider than hip distance apart, pulling down toward the mat.

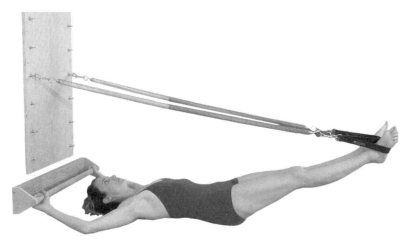

3. Inhale

Pull heels together at the bottom of the circle. Then lift legs up to starting position.

Repeat 4 times then reverse directions.

LEG SPRINGS SET UP

- 2nd–4th eyebolt from the floor
- Adjust 1–2 eyebolts higher if you have a newer Springboard that goes up to 10 or 11

FUNCTIONS & TARGET MUSCLES

- Strengthens hamstrings, external rotators and adductors
- Abdominals and deep spinal muscles stabilize pelvis and spine while hip moves through wide ROM
- Teaches disassociation of the femur from the pelvis as hips move in multiple planes

ALIGNMENT CUES & OBSTACLES

- ROM is greater in turn out—leg circles will be bigger than rectangles
- Feel femurs wrapping around to outside of legs to increase and maintain external rotation of hip
- If client has unstable pelvis, keep ROM small when working in turn out
- Focus on moving from the top of the femur—closer to the body's center than the feet
- Keep heels together and knees straight when moving up and down center line, inner thighs pulling together—when heels are together the knee joint cannot hyperextend

VARIATIONS & PEEL BACKS

- **Variation:** *Medial Rotation Ovals*—when hip joint is rotated inward, the ROM will be more like ovals than circles
- **Peel Backs:** *Leg Pulls* and *Open/Close*

IMAGINE...*you are inscribing circles with your toes.*

ELLIE SAYS...*"This lubricates your hip joints!"*

LEG SPRINGS SET UP

- 2nd–4th eyebolt from the floor
- Adjust 1–2 eyebolts higher if you have a newer Springboard that goes up to 10 or 11

FUNCTIONS & TARGET MUSCLES

- Strengthens adductors, quads, hamstrings and external hip rotators
- Challenges abdominals to maintain neutral spine while legs are in motion
- Peel back for *Dolphin*

ALIGNMENT CUES & OBSTACLES

- Keep legs at consistent angle—no wavering up and down
- Don't snap knees straight; keep heels together to prevent knee hyperextension
- Don't let hips roll to parallel when knees straighten—use the low glutes to maintain external rotation of the hip
- Keep knees outside of springs and, if springs are banging into knees, raise legs

VARIATIONS & PEEL BACKS

- Can perform *Frogs* with parallel legs, knees and ankles touching

IMAGINE…*you have laser beams shooting out your heels every time the legs straighten.*

ELLIE SAYS…*"Frogs with leg springs is considerably more difficult than Frogs on the Reformer."*

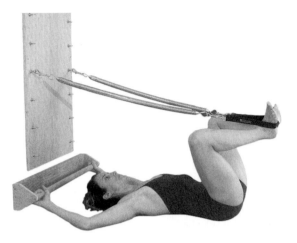

1. Starting Position — *5 to 8 repetitions in each direction*
Place feet in loops. Legs in a "frog squat" with hips in external rotation, feet flexed with heels together.

Inhale to prepare

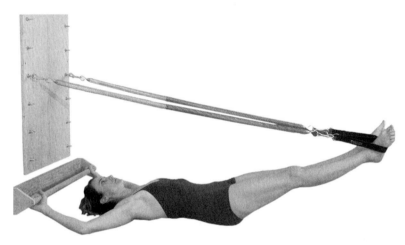

2. Exhale
Feel abdominals pulling toward spine while pressing through the heels as legs straighten on a diagonal (about 45 degrees). Maintain heel connection and neutral spine.

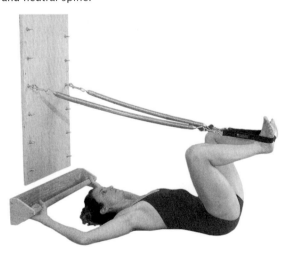

3. Inhale
Return to "frog squat" without flexing lumbar spine and losing neutral.

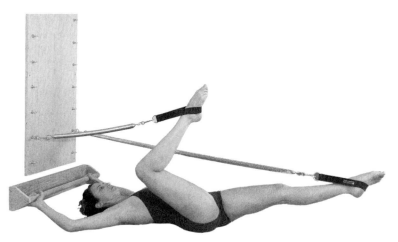

1. Starting Position — *3 to 5 repetitions in each direction*
Feet in loops. Legs extended in external rotation. Bend one leg in toward your body, as the other leg reaches long and away.

Inhale to prepare

LEG SPRINGS SET UP
- 2nd–4th eyebolt from the floor
- Adjust 1–2 eyebolts higher if you have a newer Springboard that goes up to 10 or 11

FUNCTIONS & TARGET MUSCLES
- Strengthens adductors, quads, hamstrings and external hip rotators
- Challenges abdominals to maintain neutral spine with legs in motion

ALIGNMENT CUES & OBSTACLES
- Feel the length in the front of the hips as you reach the legs long away from you
- Keep knees outside of springs and if springs are banging into knees, raise legs

IMAGINE...*you are riding along the English countryside.*

ELLIE SAYS...*"This exercise is awkward, but after you get the hang of it...fun."*

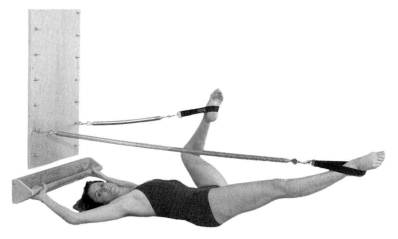

2. Breathing continuously
Circle the bent leg up and diagonally away, as if pushing a pedal on a bicycle, keeping knee just outside of spring. Alternate legs in the bicycle movement, reaching long through the heels as you extend the legs diagonally forward.

Repeat 3–5 times and reverse directions.

LEG SPRINGS SET UP

- 2nd–4th eyebolt from the floor
- Adjust 1–2 eyebolts higher if you have a newer Springboard that goes up to 10 or 11

FUNCTIONS & TARGET MUSCLES

- Strengthens adductors, quads, hamstrings and external hip rotators
- Challenges abdominals to maintain neutral spine while legs are in motion

ALIGNMENT CUES & OBSTACLES

- Don't snap knees straight; keep heels together to prevent knee hyperextension
- Don't let hips roll to parallel when knees straighten—use the low glutes
- Keep knees outside of springs and if springs are banging into knees, raise legs

VARIATIONS & PEEL BACKS

- **Peel Back:** *Frog Extensions*

IMAGINE...*your legs are a dolphin's tail propelling you through the ocean.*

ELLIE SAYS...*"Dolphin is a 'circular frog', combining a frog extension with a leg pull."*

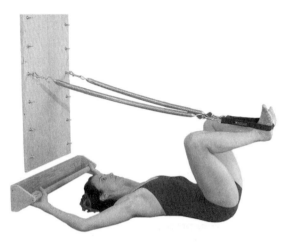

1. Starting Position — *6 to 8 repetitions*
Place feet in loops. Legs in a "frog squat" with hips in external rotation, feet flexed with heels together.

Inhale to prepare

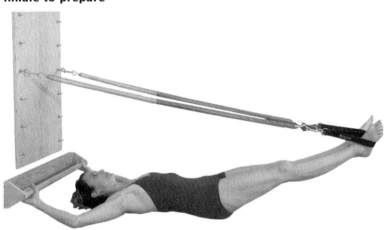

2. Exhale
Feel abdominals pulling toward spine; press through the heels as legs straighten on a diagonal (about 45 degrees). Maintain heel connection and neutral spine.

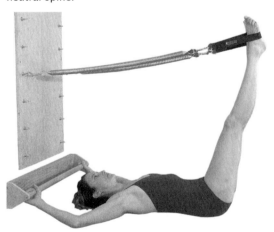

3. Inhale
Keeping legs together, raise legs to the starting position of your "leg pull" (about 90 degrees) and then pull the legs down into a frog squat (starting position).

Repeat sequence 3–4 times and reverse directions:
From frog squat, straighten knees and reach legs up to the sky, then pull legs down to 45 degrees, and return to the frog squat (starting position).

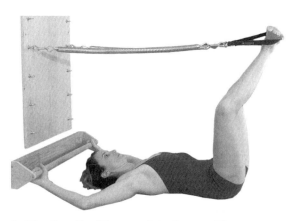

1. Starting Position — *4 to 8 repetitions*
Feet in straps with heels together, feet flexed, hips externally rotated and in flexion with knees bent open into a diamond shape.

Inhale to prepare

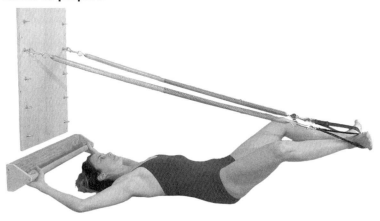

2. Exhale
Scoop abdominals and pull legs down toward mat while keeping pelvis and spine neutral. Think of opening knee to initiate the pull.

3. Inhale
Control legs back to starting position.

VARIATION: Levitation (Intermediate)

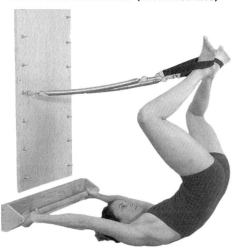

LEG SPRINGS SET UP
- 2nd–4th eyebolt from the floor
- Adjust 1–2 eyebolts higher if you have a newer Springboard that goes up to 10 or 11

FUNCTIONS & TARGET MUSCLES
- Strengthens external rotators of the hip
- Teaches disassociation of the femur from the pelvis
- Works the hamstring double duty—pulling hip into extension and flexing the knee—and triple duty for biceps femoris, the lateral hamstring, since it aids in external rotation of hip
- Peel back for *Dolphin*

ALIGNMENT CUES & OBSTACLES
- Leg position is halfway between *Frog Squat* position and straight legs
- Initiate pull from underneath the leg
- Open the knees from the back of the hip and feel the wrapping sensation around the top of the thighs
- Keep pelvis stable while initiating leg pull—it is really easy to tuck pelvis with hips in external rotation

VARIATIONS & PEEL BACKS
- **Modification:** Keep ROM small if client cannot maintain pelvic stability
- **Variation:** *Diamond Pulls with Levitation* (Intermediate): First press arms straight, reaching body away from bar. Pull legs in diamond shape down toward mat. Exhale and engage glutes and levitate pelvis maintaining diamond shape of legs. Repeat up and down motion hinging from upper back. **Contraindications:** Disc dysfunction, osteoporosis, neck problems

IMAGINE...*you're moving your legs from the "panty line" muscles contracting.*

ELLIE SAYS...*"This is a great exercise for creating that "high butt" we often use as a selling point of Pilates."*

LEVITATED DOLPHIN

LEG SPRINGS SET UP

- 2nd–4th eyebolt from the floor
- Adjust 1–2 eyebolts higher if you have a newer Springboard that goes up to 10 or 11

FUNCTIONS & TARGET MUSCLES

- Strengthens adductors, quads, hamstrings, glutes and external hip rotators

ALIGNMENT CUES & OBSTACLES

- Don't snap knees straight; keep heels together to prevent knee hyperextension
- Keep knees outside of springs; if springs are banging into knees, raise legs
- Makes sure shoulders stay stabilized down away from the ears—widen the arms if you are unable to keep shoulders down
- If you feel tension in your neck or upper traps, bend the elbows and stabilize with bent arms instead of straight arms
- **Contraindications:** Disc dysfunction, osteoporosis, neck problems

VARIATIONS & PEEL BACKS

- **Peel Back:** *Dolphin Without Levitation*

IMAGINE...*a hot spatula lifts your butt perkily off the mat in levitation.*

ELLIE SAYS...*"Dolphin with Levitation is similar to Short Spine Stretch on the Reformer."*

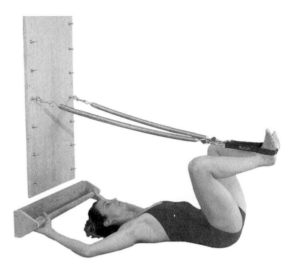

1. Starting Position — *6 to 8 repetitions*
Lie supine, hold onto the foot bar and press long away from the Springboard with your arms. Place feet in loops. Legs are in a "frog squat" with hips in external rotation, feet flexed with heels together.

Inhale to prepare

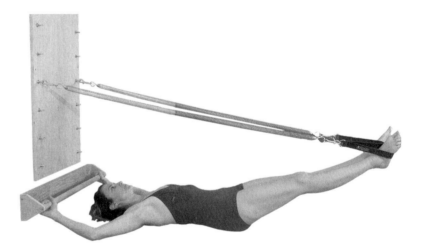

2. Exhale
Feel abdominals pulling toward spine; press through the heels as legs straighten on a diagonal (about 45 degrees). Maintain heel connection and neutral spine.

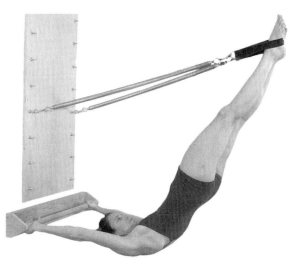

3. Inhale
Squeeze inner thighs together and levitate your hips up, lifting your legs up to the sky. (You will come out of resistance at the top, so you must maintain the levitation with your powerhouse muscles).

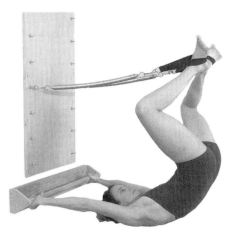

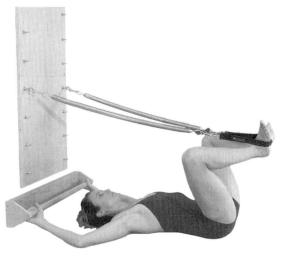

4. Exhale
Peel down your spine one vertebra at a time as you pull the legs down into a frog squat (starting position).

Repeat sequence 3–4 times and reverse directions:
From frog squat, reach legs up to the sky, levitating hips off the mat, then leg pull down to 45 degrees, allowing the butt to land on the mat and return to *Frog* squat position.

LEG SPRINGS SET UP

- 4th–9th eyebolt from the floor
- Adjust 1–2 eyebolts higher if you have a newer Springboard that goes up to 10 or 11

FUNCTIONS & TARGET MUSCLES

- Teaches total levitation
- Deeply strengthens the "powerhouse" hamstrings, glutes, inner thighs and core

ALIGNMENT CUES & OBSTACLES

- Don't attempt with a client who is not strong enough to maintain a perfect plank in the air—you can injure the neck or the lower back!
- Spot client by putting hands under their heels when their legs are close to the floor and their back is still in contact with the mat. Have them press their heels down into your hands to initiate the levitation. The extension of the hip should lift the whole body up into the plank. If the hips flex at all, the client either is not ready to do this series, or needs heavier resistance.
- Feel legs lengthen away from torso as torso lengthens away from legs (opposing energy helps to create stability)
- Keep feet relaxed—neither pointed nor flexed
- **Obstacles:** Acute phase of hamstring pull, strain, or tear; neck problems
- **Contraindications:** Disc dysfunction, osteoporosis, neck problems

VARIATIONS & PEEL BACKS

- **Peel Back:** *Double Leg Spring*s
- Can also be done with legs in parallel

IMAGINE...*a hot spatula under your butt perkily lifts your hips up to the sky!*

ELLIE SAYS...*"One of the best series to tone the butt and legs!"*

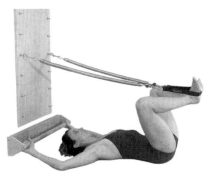

1. Starting Position — *4 to 8 repetitions*
Straps around arches of feet, hips externally rotated so feet are in Pilates "V"—keep heels together and knees straight (if heels are together knee joint cannot hyperextend), pull inner thighs together. Start in Frog squat

Inhale to prepare

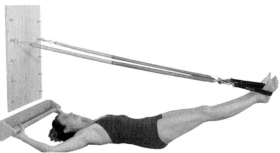

2. Exhale
Engage abdominal scoop and extend legs diagonally forward a few inches from the floor.

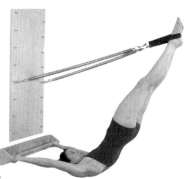

3. Inhale
Squeeze glutes to lift hips and levitate the whole body off the floor, maintaining a perfect plank and rising up as high as you can—but never onto your neck.

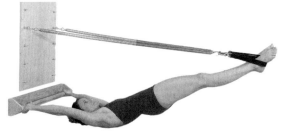

4. Exhale
Pull your whole body back down toward the floor without actually touching down, maintaining the perfect plank. Think of reaching your toes long away from you, so that your whole body is completely layed out.

Repeat steps 3–4 with 4 to 8 repetitions
Continue on with variations or come back down to mat by rolling down one vertebrae at a time.

VARIATION: Scissors

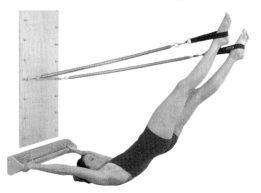

- **Variations:** *Scissors*
- **Variations:** *Running*
- **Variations:** *Bicycle*
- **Variations:** *Parallel*
- **Variations:** *Turned Out*
- **Variations:** *Circles*

- See Supine Leg Series for specific alignment details

VARIATION: Running

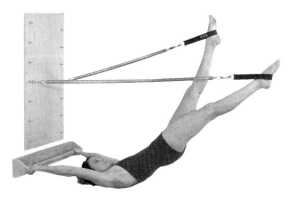

VARIATION: Bicycle

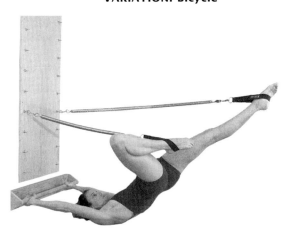

VARIATION: Circles

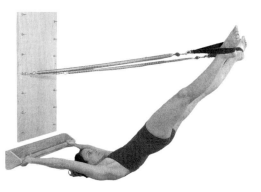

LEG SPRINGS SET UP

- 1st–3rd eyebolt from the floor
- Adjust 1–2 eyebolts higher if you have a newer Springboard that goes up to 10 or 11

FUNCTIONS & TARGET MUSCLES

- Teaches torso stability while the legs move
- Strengthens hip adductors, hamstrings, glutes, abdominals

ALIGNMENT CUES & OBSTACLES

- Keep your torso stable as your leg moves freely

VARIATIONS & PEEL BACKS

- **Modification:** Lie with head resting on bottom folded arm or small pillow to keep neck and spine in neutral position, especially for people with neck issues
- **Variation:** *Bottom Leg Up*
  Hold top leg up, a little higher than the hip, and bring the bottom leg up to meet it. Repeat 8–10 times
- **Peel Back:** *Up/Down in Parallel* on the mat

IMAGINE...*your hip is reaching long away from the ribcage.*

ELLIE SAYS...*"Great for finding your gluteus medius."*

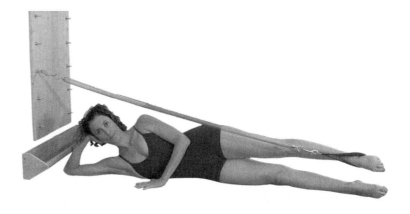

1. Starting Position — *5 to 8 repetitions*
Lie on your side, supported by your elbow, close to the springboard, with leg spring in front of your body. Place top foot in loop around arch of foot, legs in parallel, extended in line with your body.

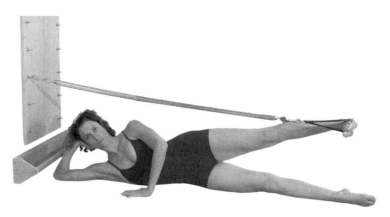

2. Inhale
Lift top leg up to the height of the hip.

3. Exhale
Flex foot and reach heel away from body as you bring the leg down.

Repeat and alternate the foot position at the top: next time point the foot at the top and bring it down.

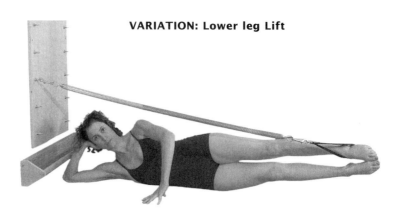

VARIATION: Lower leg Lift

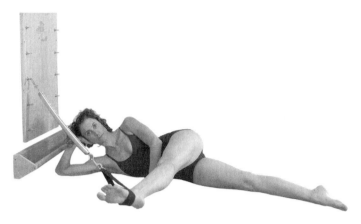

1. Starting Position — *8 to 10 repetitions*
Lie on your side with head close to the Springboard, with leg spring in front of your body. Rest your head on your bottom hand, propped on your bent elbow on the mat. Press hand of top arm into mat to help stabilize torsos. Put loop around the arch of your top foot and with legs in a Pilates "V" move them slightly in front of your body, creasing at the hip joint. Your bottom foot acts as a "kickstand" with the toes pressing onto the floor and the heel off the mat.

2. Inhale
Engage abdominal scoop and kick the leg forward, flexing the foot and gently pulsing it once to test your stability.

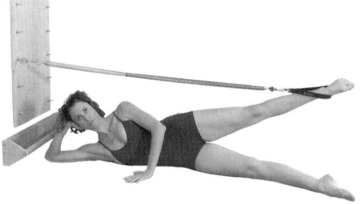

3. Exhale
Deepen your abdominal scoop and squeeze your glutes to maintain your stability as you kick the leg behind you with pointed foot, pulsing it once to test your stability.

LEG SPRINGS SET UP
- 1st–3rd eyebolt from the floor
- Adjust 1–2 eyebolts higher if you have a newer Springboard that goes up to 10 or 11

FUNCTIONS & TARGET MUSCLES
- Teaches torso stability while the leg moves forward and back
- Strengthens hip adductors, hamstrings, glutes and abdominals.

ALIGNMENT CUES & OBSTACLES
- Keep your torso stable as your leg moves freely
- Prepare your core for the back kick—think powerhouse (abdominal scoop and butt squeeze creating a posterior pelvic tilt)
- Keep your leg movements to the back small: ROM of the hip in extension is only 15 degrees—if you kick too far behind you, your spine will be extending, not your hip
- Maintain external rotation—especially when the leg is behind you!
- Keep abdominals engaged to maintain side lying neutral—bottom waist up and lifted with hips level

VARIATIONS & PEEL BACKS
- **Modification:** If client has neck issues, have them place their head on their bottom arm or place a small pillow or towel under their head
- **Variation:** *Side Kicks* can also be done in parallel
- **Peel Back:** *Side Kicks* on the mat

IMAGINE...*your torso is a plank and your leg swings freely from that stable place.*

ELLIE SAYS...*"Sharon Stone likes this series."*

LEG SPRINGS SET UP

- 1st–3rd eyebolt from the floor
- Adjust 1–2 eyebolts higher if you have a newer Springboard that goes up to 10 or 11

FUNCTIONS & TARGET MUSCLES

- Teaches torso stability while the leg moves
- Strengthens hip adductors, hamstrings, glutes, and abdominals

ALIGNMENT CUES & OBSTACLES

- Keep your torso stable as your leg moves freely
- Prepare your core for the arabesque part of the circle—think powerhouse (abdominal scoop and butt squeeze creating a posterior pelvic tilt)
- Keep your leg movements to the back small: ROM of the hip in extension is only 15 degrees—if you kick too far behind you, your spine will be extending, not your hip
- Keep abdominals engaged to maintain side lying neutral—bottom waist up and lifted with hips level

VARIATIONS & PEEL BACKS

- **Modification:** If client has neck issues, have them place their head on their bottom arm or place a small pillow or towel under their head
- *Hamstring Stretch:* Hold the leg as it reaches in front of you—pull it in toward your chest for a hamstring stretch
- *Hip Flexor Stretch:* Reach the leg behind you, bend your knee and let the spring pull you into a stretch. Hold the torso and pelvis stable by engaging your abdominal scoop and squeezing your butt, trying to tilt your pelvis posteriorly.

IMAGINE...you are drawing semi circles with your foot.

ELLIE SAYS..."This one is just more great glute workout."

VARIATION: Hip Flexor Stretch

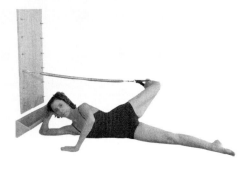

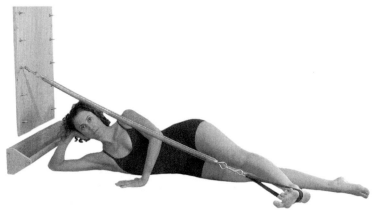

1. Starting Position — *3 to 5 repetitions*

Lie on your side with head close to the Springboard, with leg spring in front of your body. Rest your head on your bottom hand, propped on your bent elbow on the mat. Press hand of top arm into mat to help stabilize torsos. Put loop around the arch of your top foot and with legs in a Pilates "V" move them slightly in front of your body, creasing at the hip joint. Your bottom foot acts as a "kickstand" with the toes pressing onto the floor and the heel off the mat.

Inhale to prepare

Reach the top leg forward.

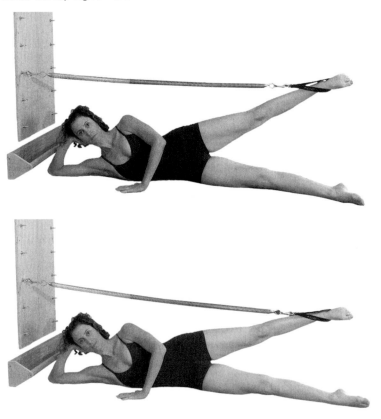

2. Exhale

Lift the leg up to the side, making an arc as you bring the leg behind you.

Repeat 3–5 times and reverse the movement, starting with reaching the leg behind you.

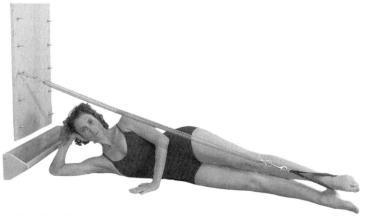

1. Starting Position — *8 to 10 repetitions*

Lie on your side with head close to the Springboard, with leg spring in front of your body. Rest your head on your bottom hand, propped on your bent elbow on the mat. Press hand of top arm into mat to help stabilize torso. Put loop around the arch of your top foot and with legs in a Pilates "V" move them slightly in front of your body, creasing at the hip joint. Your bottom foot acts as a "kickstand" with the toes pressing onto the floor and the heel off the mat.

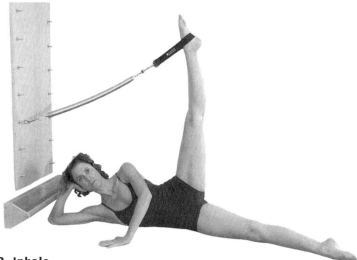

2. Inhale

Kick the leg up to the sky, maintaining external rotation.

3. Exhale

Flex the foot at the top, and then bring the leg back down to the starting position, thinking of pressing something down with your inner thigh.

VARIATION: Developé

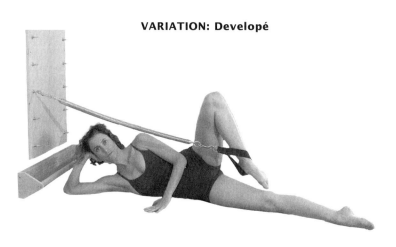

LEG SPRINGS SET UP

- 1st–3rd eyebolt from the floor
- Adjust 1–2 eyebolts higher if you have a newer Springboard that goes up to 10 or 11

FUNCTIONS & TARGET MUSCLES

- Teaches torso stability while the leg moves to the side
- Strengthens hip adductors, hamstrings, glutes, abdominals

ALIGNMENT CUES & OBSTACLES

- Keep your torso stable as your leg moves freely
- Try to reach long out of your hip as you bring the leg down
- Even though you are kicking to the side, the leg should remain towards the front of the body
- Lower the leg slowly—resist gravity and go for control
- Kick as high as you can, but just move from the hip socket and not your back

VARIATIONS & PEEL BACKS

- **Modification:** If client has neck issues, have them place their head on their bottom arm or place a small pillow or towel under their head.
- **Variation:** *Developé*: Bring your leg into passé (drawing your big toe up the inner leg until the toe reaches the inside of the knee—keep knee facing up), and then straighten the knee reaching the foot to the sky (thigh shouldn't lower as your straighten your knee). Flex your foot at the top and bring the leg back to starting position. Repeat 3 times and reverse directions.
- **Peel Back:** *Up/Down in Turned Out* on the mat

IMAGINE...*you are kicking with the Rockettes!*

ELLIE SAYS..."*Fun, fun, fun!*"

RONDE DE JAMBE

LEG SPRINGS SET UP

- 1st –3rd eyebolt from the floor
- Adjust 1–2 eyebolts higher if you have a newer Springboard that goes up to 10 or 11

FUNCTIONS & TARGET MUSCLES

- Teaches torso stability while the leg moves in large ROM
- Strengthens hip adductors, hamstrings, glutes, and abdominals

ALIGNMENT CUES & OBSTACLES

- Keep your torso stable as your leg moves freely
- Prepare your core for the arabesque part of the circle—think powerhouse (abdominal scoop and butt squeeze creating a posterior pelvic tilt)
- Keep your leg movements to the back small: ROM of the hip in extension is only 15 degrees—if you kick too far behind you, your spine will be extending, not your hip
- Maintain external rotation throughout the motion. Hint: external rotation is most available in the second position (leg up to the sky) and least available in hip extension. So you really must work the rotators when the leg is in front and behind you!

VARIATIONS & PEEL BACKS

- **Modification:** If client has neck issues, have them place their head on their bottom arm or place a small pillow or towel under their head.
- **Peel Back:** *Grande Ronde de Jambe* on the mat

IMAGINE…*someone is holding your ankle and pulling your leg out of the hip socket, making the leg oh-so-light!*

ELLIE SAYS…*"Grande Ronde de Jambe is a ballet term meaning big circle of the leg—so circle that leg and feel the work in the glutes and hips."*

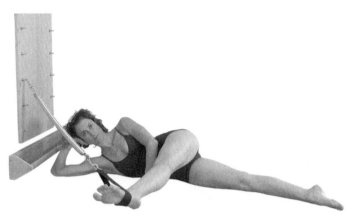

1. Starting Position — *8 to 10 repetitions*
Lie on your side with head close to the Springboard, with leg spring in front of your body. Rest your head on your bottom hand, propped on your bent elbow on the mat. Press hand of top arm into mat to help stabilize torso. Put loop around the arch of your top foot and with legs in a Pilates "V" move them slightly in front of your body, creasing at the hip joint. Your bottom foot acts as a "kickstand" with the toes pressing onto the floor and the heel off the mat.

2. Inhale
Reach the leg forward, slowly bring it up to the sky, maintaining external rotation.

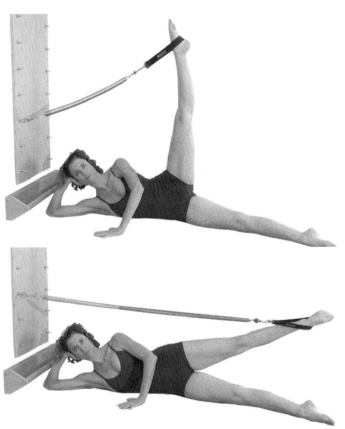

3. Exhale
Continue the circle of the leg bringing it behind you, engaging your abdominal scoop and squeezing your glutes to maintain your pelvic stability. In the arabesque position, think of bringing the top of your pelvis slightly forward to compensate for the weight of the leg behind you.

After 4 repetitions, reverse the direction of the circle and start by bringing the leg behind you, circling it up to the side, then lowering the leg in front of you.

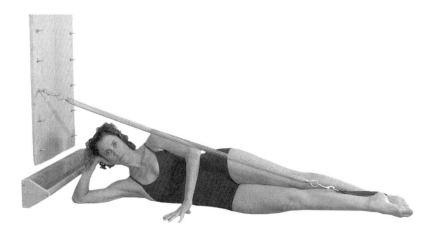

1. Starting Position — *8 to 10 repetitions*
Lie on your side with head close to the Springboard, with the leg spring in front of your body. Rest your head on your bottom hand, propped on your bent elbow on the mat. Press hand of top arm into mat to help stabilize torso. Put loop around the arch of your top foot and with legs in a Pilates "V" move them slightly in front of your body, creasing at the hip joint. Breathe continuously as you scissor the legs by bringing the top foot back and bottom foot up.

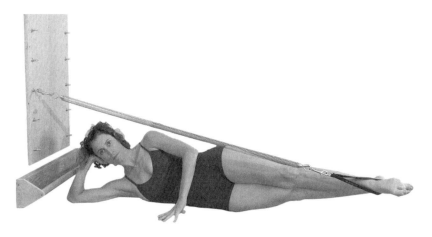

2. Switch the scissor in a small precise movement. Lift the top leg slightly up and forward, and then circle down, making a small circle in the front of the bottom leg.

Alternate scissors 6–8 more times.

LEG SPRINGS SET UP
- 1st–3rd eyebolt from the floor
- Adjust 1–2 eyebolts higher if you have a newer Springboard that goes up to 10 or 11

FUNCTIONS & TARGET MUSCLES
- Teaches torso stability while the leg moves to the side
- Strengthens hip adductors, hamstrings, glutes, abdominals

ALIGNMENT CUES & OBSTACLES
- Keep your torso stable as your leg moves freely
- Prepare your core for the arabesque part of the circle—think powerhouse (abdominal scoop and butt squeeze creating a posterior pelvic tilt
- Keep your leg movements to the back small, for ROM of the hip in extension is only 15 degrees—if you kick too far behind you, your spine will be extending, not your hip
- Maintain external rotation throughout the figure 8. Hint: external rotation is most available in the second position (leg up to the sky) and least available in hip extension. So you really must work the rotators when the leg is in front and behind you!
- Keep abdominals engaged to maintain side lying neutral—bottom waist up and lifted with hips level

VARIATIONS & PEEL BACKS
- **Modification:** If client has neck issues, have them place their head on their bottom arm or place a small pillow or towel under their head
- **Variation:** *Figure 8*
Draw a figure 8 with your top big toe going up and back, then down over bottom leg, then back up to the front and then down in the front. Repeat 4 times and reverse directions.

IMAGINE...*you are drawing Figure 8's with your big toe.*

ELLIE SAYS...*"This exercise is great for the glutes and rotators!"*

ROLL DOWN BAR

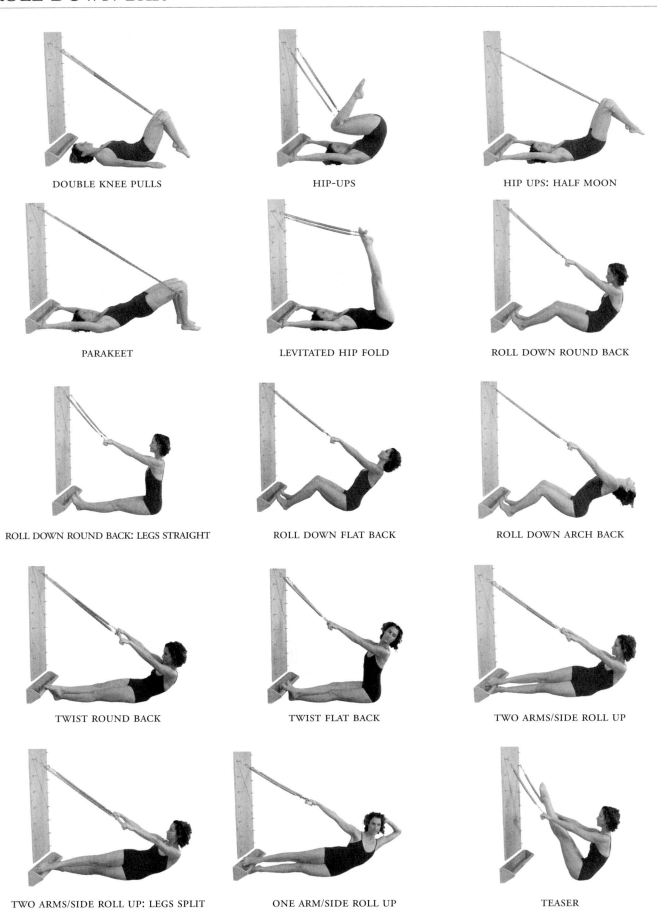

DOUBLE KNEE PULLS

HIP-UPS

HIP UPS: HALF MOON

PARAKEET

LEVITATED HIP FOLD

ROLL DOWN ROUND BACK

ROLL DOWN ROUND BACK: LEGS STRAIGHT

ROLL DOWN FLAT BACK

ROLL DOWN ARCH BACK

TWIST ROUND BACK

TWIST FLAT BACK

TWO ARMS/SIDE ROLL UP

TWO ARMS/SIDE ROLL UP: LEGS SPLIT

ONE ARM/SIDE ROLL UP

TEASER

ROLL DOWN BAR

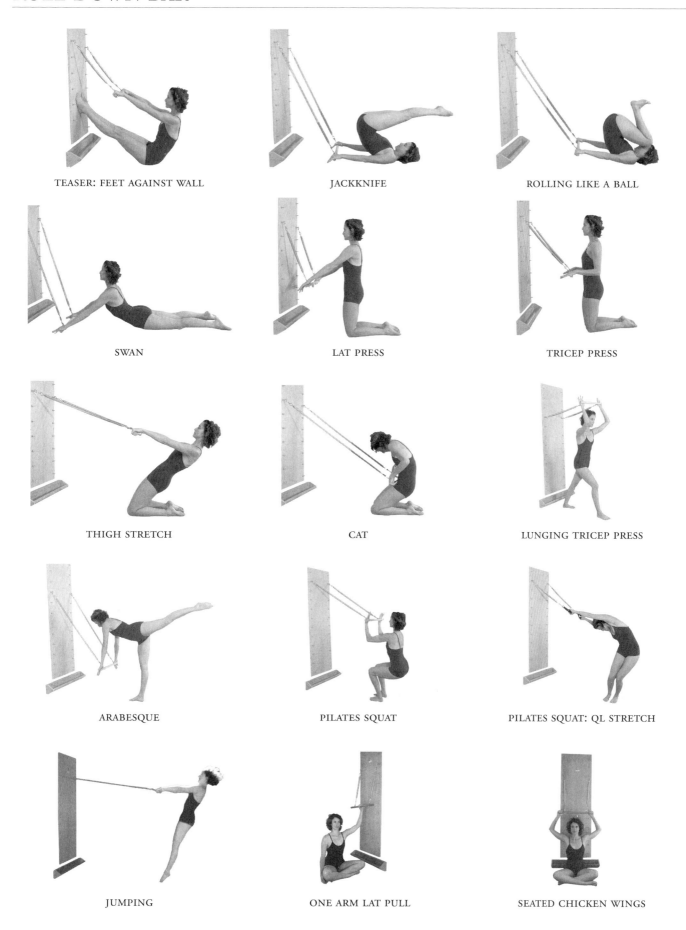

TEASER: FEET AGAINST WALL

JACKKNIFE

ROLLING LIKE A BALL

SWAN

LAT PRESS

TRICEP PRESS

THIGH STRETCH

CAT

LUNGING TRICEP PRESS

ARABESQUE

PILATES SQUAT

PILATES SQUAT: QL STRETCH

JUMPING

ONE ARM LAT PULL

SEATED CHICKEN WINGS

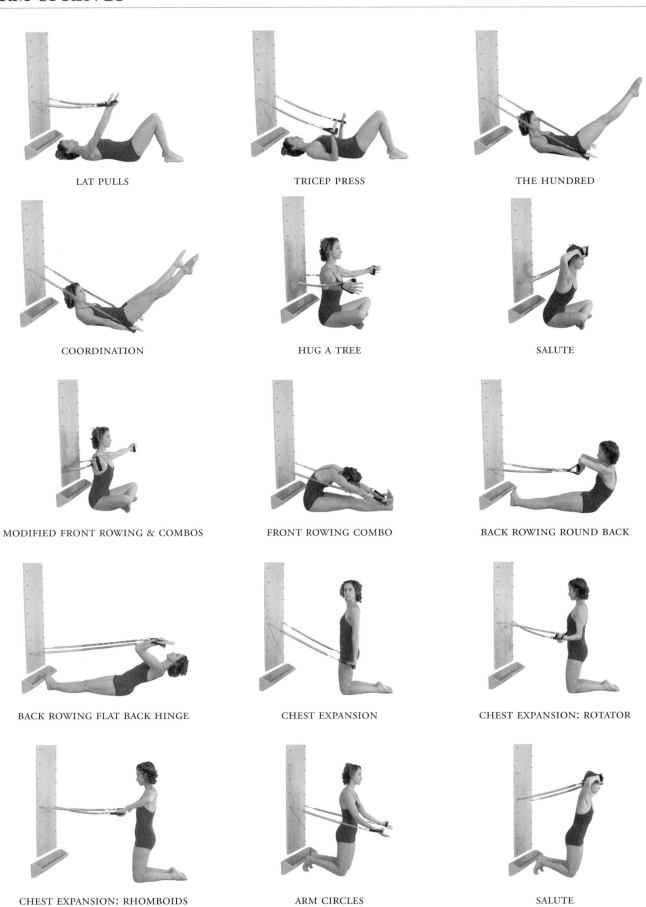

LAT PULLS

TRICEP PRESS

THE HUNDRED

COORDINATION

HUG A TREE

SALUTE

MODIFIED FRONT ROWING & COMBOS

FRONT ROWING COMBO

BACK ROWING ROUND BACK

BACK ROWING FLAT BACK HINGE

CHEST EXPANSION

CHEST EXPANSION: ROTATOR

CHEST EXPANSION: RHOMBOIDS

ARM CIRCLES

SALUTE

ARM SPRINGS

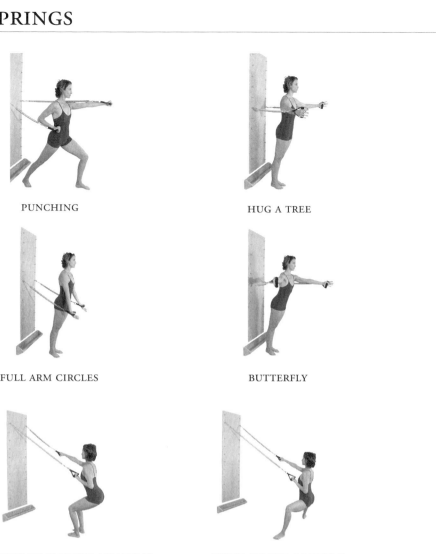

PUNCHING

HUG A TREE

SALUTE: SHAVING HEAD

FULL ARM CIRCLES

BUTTERFLY

SQUAT

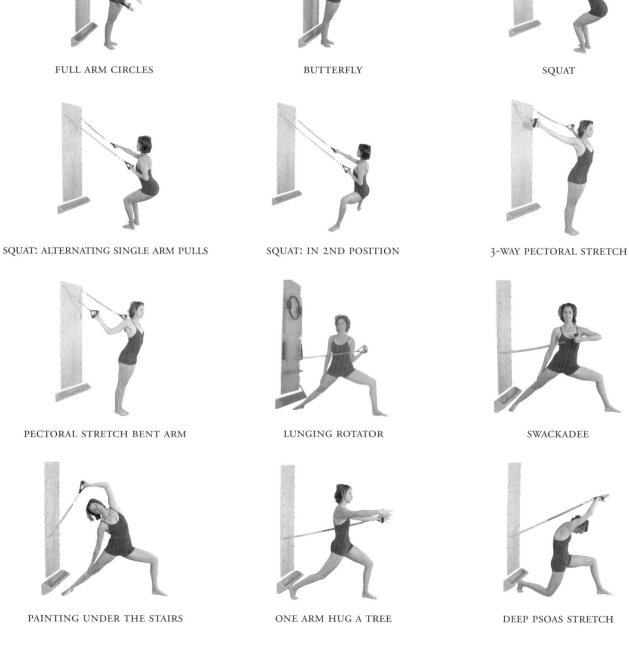

SQUAT: ALTERNATING SINGLE ARM PULLS

SQUAT: IN 2ND POSITION

3-WAY PECTORAL STRETCH

PECTORAL STRETCH BENT ARM

LUNGING ROTATOR

SWACKADEE

PAINTING UNDER THE STAIRS

ONE ARM HUG A TREE

DEEP PSOAS STRETCH

LEG SPRINGS

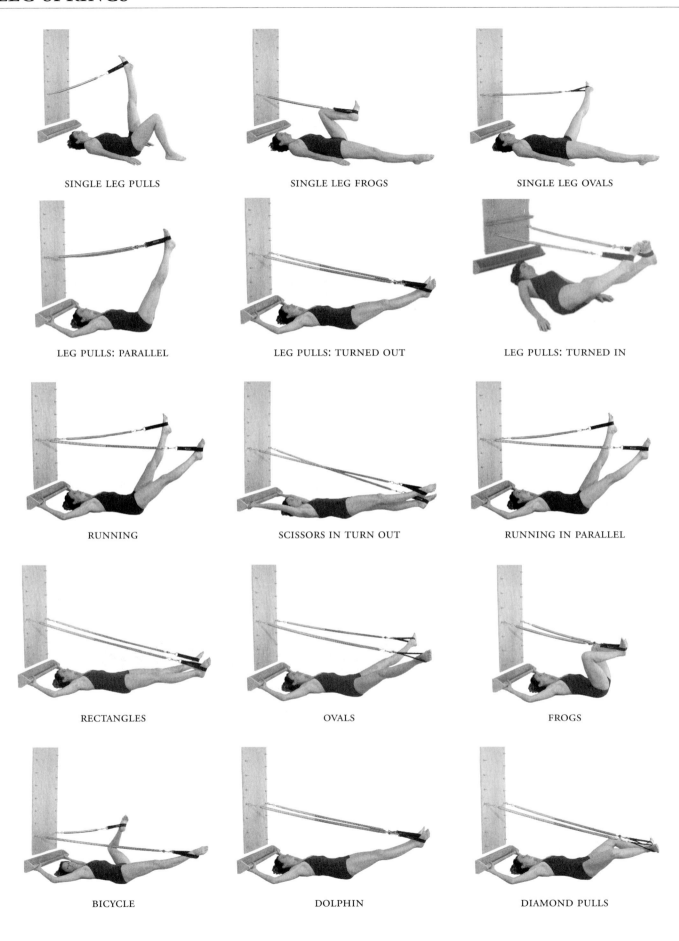

SINGLE LEG PULLS

SINGLE LEG FROGS

SINGLE LEG OVALS

LEG PULLS: PARALLEL

LEG PULLS: TURNED OUT

LEG PULLS: TURNED IN

RUNNING

SCISSORS IN TURN OUT

RUNNING IN PARALLEL

RECTANGLES

OVALS

FROGS

BICYCLE

DOLPHIN

DIAMOND PULLS

LEG SPRINGS

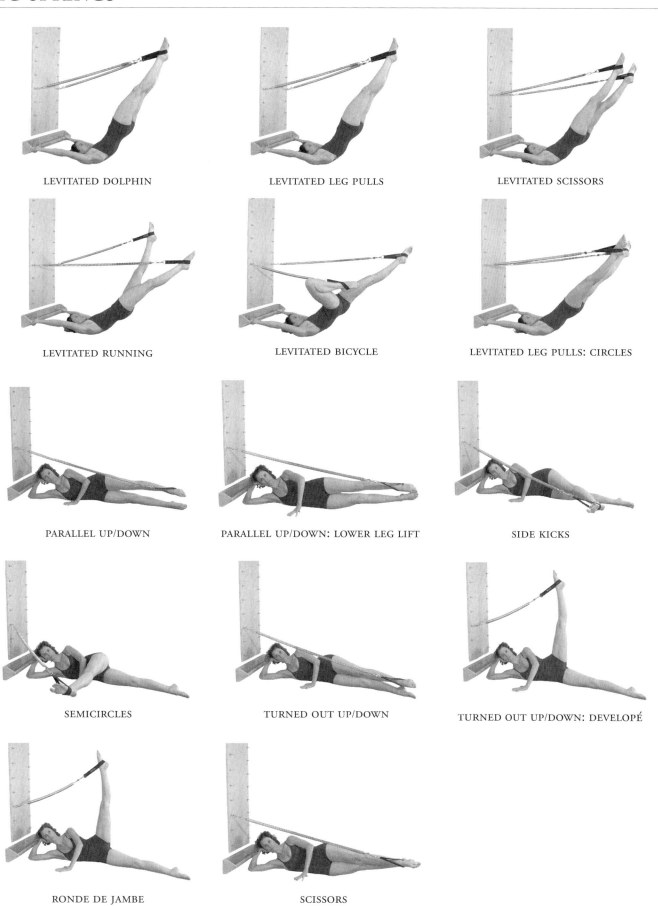

LEVITATED DOLPHIN

LEVITATED LEG PULLS

LEVITATED SCISSORS

LEVITATED RUNNING

LEVITATED BICYCLE

LEVITATED LEG PULLS: CIRCLES

PARALLEL UP/DOWN

PARALLEL UP/DOWN: LOWER LEG LIFT

SIDE KICKS

SEMICIRCLES

TURNED OUT UP/DOWN

TURNED OUT UP/DOWN: DEVELOPÉ

RONDE DE JAMBE

SCISSORS

OTHER BOOKS BY ELLIE HERMAN

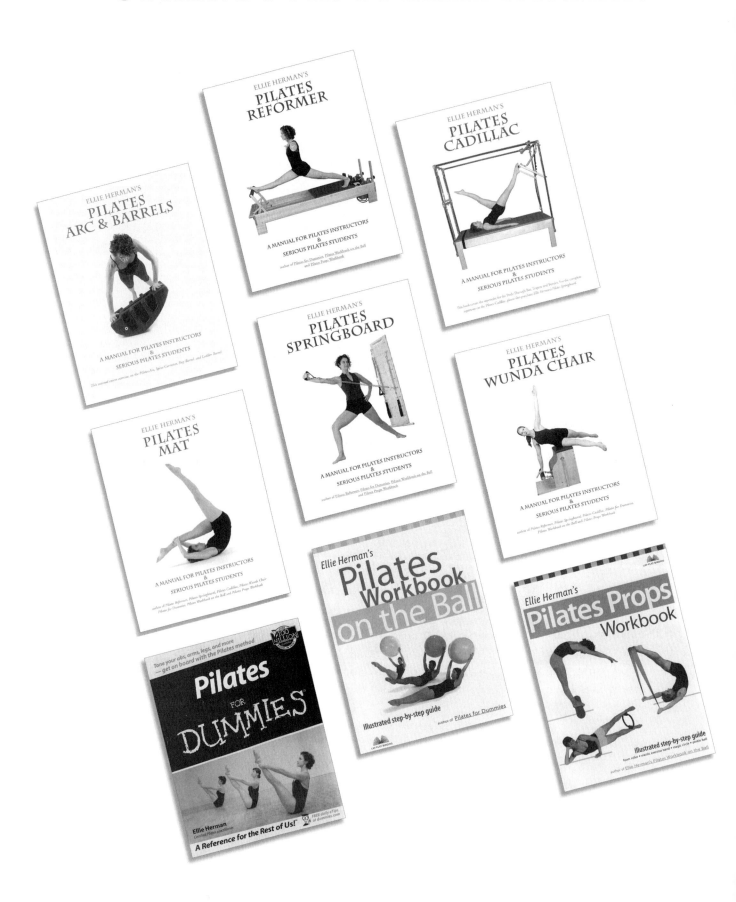

THE PILATES SPRINGBOARD
DESIGNED BY ELLIE HERMAN

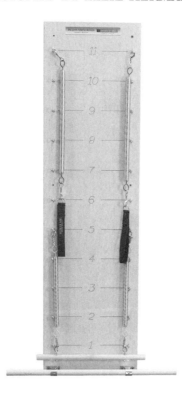

The Pilates Springboard is a space saving and affordable piece of resistance equipment which gives you a full-body workout. The Pilates Springboard consists of a 5-foot rectangular wooden board with eyebolts placed on either side at 6-inch increments and a dowel at the bottom to use for arm or foot support. It comes with:

• two arm springs with neoprene handles

• two leg springs, with cotton loops

• one wooden roll down bar

The Pilates Springboard comes with a 45-minute flow workout DVD which takes you through a warm-up, core strengthening, upper body and lower body conditioning program. Some of the exercises are from classic Pilates repertoire, and others are original exercises developed by master Pilates teacher Ellie Herman especially for the Springboard.

The Pilates Springboard is bolted into studs for support, taking up no floor space. This makes it perfect for an extra room, a home gym, garage, attic, or basement. For those with gyms or Pilates studios, you can affordably mount several Springboards along a wall and offer challenging Pilates group equipment classes without moving heavy equipment or taking up valuable storage space.

The Pilates Springboard costs $445
plus tax and shipping, and includes an instructional DVD. Purchase online from Ellie and get $25 off.
www.elliehermanpilates.com

Ellie Herman distributes **Balanced Body** Equipment. Buy any piece of
Balanced Body Equipment and receive 5–10% of your purchase price at any of our locations.
Email Ellie at **ellie@elliehermanpilates.com** for any larger purchases of **Balanced Body**.

Pilates Springboard classes offered everyday at our studios—come check them out!

ELLIE HERMAN PILATES ACADEMY

TEACHER TRAINING

Ellie believes that Pilates education begins with a deep understanding of anatomy, kinesiology, posture, and basic bio-mechanics. Ellie uses the fundamental exercises not only as an introduction to the Pilates repertoire but also as a teaching tool to reveal clients' postural habits and muscular imbalances.

Ellie is committed to teaching students the overarching applications of all the Pilates exercises, most importantly the contraindications, so that when students graduate they are confident that they can apply their Pilates knowledge to all populations. Our programs offer in-depth study of the Pilates Method with step-by-step training by a master teacher, teaching assistant opportunities to work side-by-side with a certified instructor, and a fully equipped studio available to teachers-in-training for practice and student teaching.

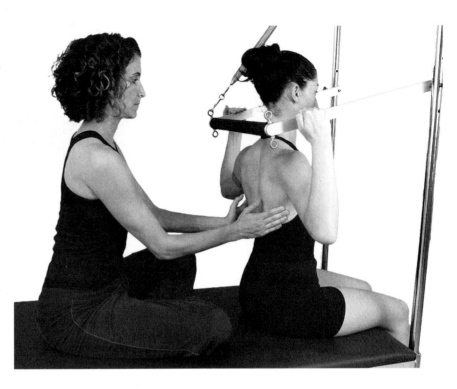

Private Pilates Certification: Ellie Herman is available in Brooklyn and specially trained instructors in Oakland are available to do Private Pilates Certification. This option is perfect for anyone who travels from abroad and needs to do their training at a specific time or anyone who can't fit the module schedule into their own.

For more information visit:
www.elliehermanpilates.com/education/teacher-training

HOST ELLIE

You can bring Ellie to your studio to teach a Pilates Teacher Training, Professional Workshops, or Public classes. Email Ellie directly to schedule **education@elliehermanpilates.com.**

For more information visit:
www.elliehermanpilates.com/education/host-ellie

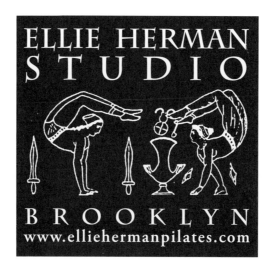

www.elliehermanpilates.com

Ellie Herman Studios distributes **Balanced Body** Equipment. Buy a Springboard or any **Balanced Body** Equipment and receive 5% of your purchase price in products or services at any of our locations.

ELLIE HERMAN STUDIO
788A Union Street
Brooklyn, NY 11215
phone: (718)230-3707
email: brooklyn@ellie.net

ELLIE HERMAN STUDIO ANNEX
463 4th St.
Brooklyn, NY 11215
phone: (718)230-3707
email: brooklyn@ellie.net

CHANGING THE WORLD ONE VERTEBRA AT A TIME

EXERCISE INDEX